Handbook of Differential Diagnosis in Neurology

Handbook of Differential Diagnosis in Neurology

Edited by

Nicholas P. Poolos, M.D., Ph.D.

Instructor of Neurology and Neuroscience,
Baylor College of Medicine, Houston;
Staff Physician, Department of Neurology,
Veterans Affairs Medical Center, Houston

with 10 contributing authors

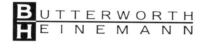

Boston Oxford Auckland Johannesburg Melbourne New Delhi

Every effort has been made to ensure that the drug dosage schedules within this text are accurate and conform to standards accepted at time of publication. However, as treatment recommendations vary in the light of continuing research and clinical experience, the reader is advised to verify drug dosage schedules herein with information found on product information sheets. This is especially true in cases of new or infrequently used drugs.

∞ Recognizing the importance of preserving what has been written, Butterworth–Heinemann prints its books on acid-free paper whenever possible.

Library of Congress Cataloging-in-Publication Data

Handbook of differential diagnosis in neurology / [edited by] Nicholas P. Poolos.
   p. ; cm.
  Includes bibliographical references and index.
  ISBN 0-7506-7002-9 (alk. paper)
   1. Nervous system—Diagnosis—Handbooks, manuals, etc. 2. Diagnosis, Differential—Handbooks, manuals, etc. 3. Neurologic examination—Handbooks, manuals, etc. I. Poolos, Nicholas P.
   [DNLM: 1. Nervous System Diseases—diagnosis—Handbooks. 2. Diagnosis, Differential—Handbooks. WL 39 H23654 2001]
  RC348 .H294 2001
  616.8'0475—dc21   00-051904

British Library Cataloguing-in-Publication Data
A catalogue record for this book is available from the British Library.

The publisher offers special discounts on bulk orders of this book.
For information, please contact:

Manager of Special Sales
Butterworth-Heinemann
225 Wildwood Avenue
Woburn, MA 01801-2041
Tel: 781-904-2500
Fax: 781-904-2620

For information on all Butterworth–Heinemann publications available, contact our World Wide Web home page at: http://www.bh.com

10 9 8 7 6 5 4 3 2 1

Printed in the United States of America

To Harriet
for her love, enthusiasm, and optimism

Contents

Contributing Authors

Kanokwan Boonyapisit, M.D.
Fellow in Neurology, Case Western Reserve University, Cleveland;
Fellow in Neurology, University Hospitals of Cleveland

Adrian J. Goldszmidt, M.D.
Instructor of Neurology, Johns Hopkins University School of Medicine,
Baltimore; Director of Cerebrovascular Program, Division of Neurology,
Department of Medicine, Sinai Hospital of Baltimore

George J. Hutton, M.D.
Instructor of Neurology, Baylor College of Medicine, Houston

Cheryl A. Jay, M.D.
Associate Clinical Professor of Neurology, University of California,
San Francisco, School of Medicine; Attending Neurologist, San Francisco
General Hospital

Henry J. Kaminski, M.D.
Associate Professor of Neurology and Neurosciences, Case Western
Reserve University, Cleveland; Staff Physician, Department of Neurology,
Veterans Affairs Medical Center, University Hospitals of Cleveland

Joseph D. Pinter, M.D.
Assistant Professor of Neurology and Pediatrics, University of Washington
School of Medicine, Seattle; Staff Neurologist, Department of Neurology,
Children's Hospital and Regional Medical Center, Seattle

Nicholas P. Poolos, M.D., Ph.D.
Instructor of Neurology and Neuroscience, Baylor College of Medicine,
Houston; Staff Physician, Department of Neurology, Veterans Affairs
Medical Center, Houston

Jong M. Rho, M.D.
Assistant Professor of Pediatrics, University of California, Irvine,
College of Medicine

George M. Ringholz, M.D., Ph.D.
Chief of Behavioral Neurology and Neuropsychology, and Assistant
Professor of Neurology, Baylor College of Medicine, Houston

Ericka P. Simpson, M.D.
Assistant Professor of Neurology, Baylor College of Medicine, Houston;
Staff Physician, Department of Neurology, Ben Taub Hospital, Houston

Matthew D. Troyer, M.D.
Adjunct Instructor of Neurology, University of California, San Francisco,
School of Medicine

Preface

Differential diagnosis is difficult. This is not the clinician's fault. Throughout medical school and residency, we generally are taught a disease-oriented approach to medicine, learning the characteristics of individual syndromes. But, in practice, few patients arrive with a diagnosis stamped on their forehead—instead they present with signs and symptoms. A diagnosis must be arrived at, sometimes with difficulty, by working backward to match clinical presentation with a list of possible causes. Nowhere is this process more complicated than in neurology.

I assembled this book with the hope of making the process a little easier. My aim has been to provide succinct, one-page differentials for a variety of common neurological presentations, all with just enough descriptive annotation to allow the reader to understand how to choose among the possibilities. Clinical pearls are sprinkled throughout. And the emphasis is firmly on the most frequently encountered disease entities and presentations, with the zebras clearly labeled and herded away from the horses. I would recommend reading this book slowly, skipping from one page to another, gradually assembling an armamentarium of differentials. You will soon be better prepared for that inevitable bone-chilling moment when your attending or board examiner says, "So, what are the causes of third nerve palsy?"

Nicholas P. Poolos
Houston, Texas

Acknowledgments

I would like to thank the contributors to this book, each of whom has generously provided outstanding material in his or her field of expertise.

Thanks to my colleagues who critically commented on sections of the manuscript: Richard Hrachovy, M.D.; Hazem Machkas, M.D.; William Ondo, M.D.; Pete Poolos, M.D.; Michael Ronthal, M.D.; Paul Schulz, M.D.; and Stephen Waxman, M.D., Ph.D.

Thanks to Susan Pioli of Butterworth-Heinemann for her patience and sage advice.

My greatest debt of gratitude is owed to my wife, Harriet Saxe, for her support throughout this project. To her I dedicate this volume.

Common Abbreviations

ACA: anterior cerebral artery
ACE: angiotensin converting enzyme
ACTH: adrenocorticotropic hormone
AED: antiepileptic drug
AD: autosomal dominant
AFB: acid-fast bacilli
AIDS: acquired immunodeficiency syndrome
ALS: amyotrophic lateral sclerosis
ANA: antinuclear antibodies
ANCA: antineutrophil cytoplasmic antibodies
AR: autosomal recessive
ASD: atrial septal defect
AVM: arteriovenous malformation
BBB: blood-brain barrier
BP: blood pressure
CADASIL: cerebral autosomal dominant arteriopathy with subcortical
    infarcts and leukoencephalopathy
CBC: complete blood count
CBZ: carbamazepine
CIDP: chronic inflammatory demyelinating polyneuropathy
CK: creatine kinase
CMAP: compound muscle action potential
CMT: Charcot-Marie-Tooth disease
CN: cranial nerve
CNS: central nervous system
CP: complex partial (seizure)
CSF: cerebrospinal fluid
CT: computed tomography
CXR: chest X-ray
ds-DNA: double-stranded DNA
DM: diabetes mellitus
EEG: electroencephalogram
EM: electron microscopy
EMG: electromyogram
ESR: erythrocyte sedimentation rate

EtOH: alcohol
ETX: ethosuximide
FLAIR: fluid-attenuated inversion recovery (imaging)
GBS: Guillain-Barré syndrome
GI: gastrointestinal
GTC: generalized tonic-clonic (seizure)
HIV: human immunodeficiency virus
HMSN: hereditary motor and sensory neuropathy
HSV: Herpes simplex virus
HTLV-1: human T-cell lymphotropic virus type 1
HTN: hypertension
ICU: intensive care unit
IM: intramuscular
INH: isoniazid
INO: internuclear ophthalmoplegia
IV: intravenous
IVIG: intravenous immunoglobulin
LMN: lower motor neuron
LP: lumbar puncture
MCA: middle cerebral artery
MD: muscular dystrophy
MGUS: monoclonal gammopathy of undetermined significance
MI: myocardial infarction
MRI: magnetic resonance imaging
MS: multiple sclerosis
NCS: nerve conduction studies
NF: neurofibromatosis
NSAID: nonsteroidal antiinflammatory drug
OCB: oligoclonal band
PCA: posterior cerebral artery
PD: Parkinson's disease
PHT: phenytoin
PICA: posterior inferior cerebellar artery
PNS: peripheral nervous system
PSP: progressive supranuclear palsy
PTT: partial thromboplastin time
REM: rapid eye movement (sleep)
RF: rheumatoid factor
RPR: rapid plasma reagin
SCA: spinocerebellar ataxia
SLE: systemic lupus erythematosus
SNAP: sensory nerve action potential
SPEP: serum protein electrophoresis
SSRI: selective serotonin re-uptake inhibitor

T1 or T1WI: T1-weighted magnetic resonance imaging
T2 or T2WI: T2-weighted magnetic resonance imaging
TB: tuberculosis
TIA: transient ischemic attack
UMN: upper motor neuron
VPA: valproate
XLR: X-linked recessive

Handbook of Differential Diagnosis in Neurology

1

Common Signs and Symptoms of Neurologic Disease

Nicholas P. Poolos

LOCALIZATION

ALTERED MENTAL STATUS

CRANIAL NERVE DYSFUNCTION

Upper Motor Neuron vs. Lower Motor Neuron Weakness

Feature	UMN Lesion	LMN Lesion
Distribution	Pyramidal	Nerve root or nerve or diffuse
Movements affected	Fine, rapid movements most affected	All movements equally affected
Tone	Increased	Decreased
Reflexes	Increased	Decreased or absent
Babinski or other pathologic reflexes	Yes	No
Muscle atrophy	No	Yes
Fasciculations	No	Yes

UMN: upper motor neuron; LMN: lower motor neuron.

One of the most basic distinctions in neurological diagnosis is between lesions that cause weakness by affecting motor neurons in the central nervous system (upper motor neurons) and those in the peripheral nervous system (lower motor neurons). One principal difference is that UMN lesions will cause disproportionate weakness in so-called pyramidally innervated muscles; that is, those not involved in antigravity posture. In the upper extremities, these are the limb extensors (deltoid, triceps, wrist extensors, and interossei), while in the lower extremities these are the limb flexors (hip flexors, hamstrings, and foot dorsiflexors). UMN lesions also most affect rapid, coordinated movements, while LMN lesions affect all kinds of movement equally.

Harrison (1987).

Upper Motor Neuron vs. Lower Motor Neuron Weakness of the Face

Clinical Sign	UMN Lesion	LMN Lesion
Weakness	Muscles of lower half of face, sparing the forehead	All facial muscles, including the forehead
Long-tract signs	May be present	Absent
Facial expression	Voluntary facial expression is depressed; "emotional" facial expression is less affected	Both voluntary and "emotional" facial expression are depressed
Taste (anterior two-thirds of tongue)	Intact	May be decreased
Lacrimation, salivation	Intact	May be decreased
Corneal reflex	Normal or heightened	Depressed
Acoustic reflex	Normal	May be decreased (sounds louder on affected side)

UMN: upper motor neuron; LMN: lower motor neuron.

Acute, unilateral facial weakness is a common clinical problem. Usually, upper motor neuron causes, such as stroke, can be distinguished by history and brief examination from lower motor neuron causes, like Bell's palsy. Occasionally, it is more difficult to distinguish between the two, especially in the elderly, who may present with either. The signs shown here allow discrimination of upper motor neuron lesions from lower motor neuron lesions. A few quirks of anatomy form the basis of the most reliable signs: The frontalis muscle of the forehead has bilateral upper motor neuron innervation, so it is not affected by a unilateral UMN lesion; reflex "emotional" facial expression is localized at a brainstem nuclear level, so UMN lesions do not abolish reflex smiling (such as to a joke) as LMN lesions would.

Hanson and Sweeney (2000).

Neuropathic vs. Myopathic Weakness

Feature	Neuropathic	Myopathic
Distribution of weakness	Distal	Proximal
Reflexes	Absent	Usually present
Sensory loss	Usually present	Absent
Atrophy	Present	Absent until late
CPK	Normal	Elevated
Nerve conduction velocity	Usually decreased	Normal
EMG	Fibrillations and fasciculations	Small motor units
Muscle biopsy	Group atrophy	Irregular, necrotic fibers

Weakness due to peripheral nerve dysfunction can be distinguished from weakness due to muscle pathology by a variety of signs and laboratory tests. Among these, the most reliable signs are a proximal distribution in myopathic weakness vs. a distal distribution in neuropathic disease, the preservation of reflexes in myopathic disease, and sensory loss accompanying neuropathy. Notable exceptions to these rules include myotonic dystrophy, a muscle disease presenting with distal weakness; polymyositis, which often presents with loss of reflexes; and anterior horn cell disease, which lacks sensory loss.

Olson et al. (1994).

Lesion Localization at Different Levels of the Nervous System

Location	Weakness	Sensory Loss	Reflexes	Other Features
Cerebral cortex	UMN	Higher order	Increased	Loss of higher cognitive functions Seizures Myoclonus
Cerebral white matter and subcortical ganglia	UMN	Higher order (cerebrum); lower order (thalamus)	Increased	Loss of higher cognitive functions Psychiatric and mood disturbances Movement disorders
Brainstem	UMN	Lower order	Increased	Cranial nerve dysfunction contralateral to long-tract dysfunction
Spinal cord	UMN below lesion LMN at lesion level	Lower order	Increased	Sensory level at or below lesion Bowel/bladder dysfunction
Peripheral nerve	LMN	Lower order	Decreased	Root or nerve distribution of deficit
Neuromuscular junction	Myopathic	None	Normal	Fatiguable weakness of proximal and/or bulbar muscles
Muscle	Myopathic	None	Normal	Nonfatiguable weakness of proximal muscles

Weakness can be classified as either upper motor neuron (UMN, with spastic weakness of pyramidal distribution muscles), lower motor neuron (LMN, with flaccid weakness of muscles innervated by a given nerve), or myopathic (diffuse weakness of proximal muscles). Sensory loss can be either of lower order modalities, such as touch or temperature, or higher order functions such as stereognosis or two-point discrimination. Note that loss of lower order sensation may impair higher order sensation as well. Absent reflexes are the diagnostic hallmark of peripheral nerve disease.

Harrison (1987).

Localization of Spinal Cord Lesions

Location	Clinical Features
Craniocervical junction	Neck pain, head tilt Downbeating nystagmus UMN weakness in all four extremities
Cervical spinal cord	Neck pain Radicular signs in upper extremities at level of lesion Bilateral UMN weakness below level of lesion Sensory level at or below level of lesion Bowel/bladder dysfunction (spastic)
Thoracic spinal cord	Back pain Radicular signs at level of lesion Spastic paraparesis Sensory level below level of lesion Bowel/bladder dysfunction (spastic)
Cauda equina	Low back and perineal pain LMN weakness of lower extremities Bowel/bladder dysfunction (areflexic)
Conus medullaris	Bowel/bladder (areflexic) and sexual dysfunction Minimal lower extremity weakness Perineal sensory loss
Anterior cord syndrome	LMN weakness at level of lesion UMN weakness below lesion Loss of pain/temperature sensation below level of lesion Spared position sensation Bowel/bladder dysfunction
Central cord syndrome	Loss of pain/temperature sensation at level of lesion (suspended sensory level) UMN weakness below level of lesion Spared position sensation
Brown-Séquard syndrome (hemicord syndrome)	Ipsilateral UMN weakness below level of lesion Ipsilateral loss of position sensation below level of lesion Contralateral loss of pain/temperature sensation below level of lesion Ipsilateral loss of all sensory modalities at level of lesion

Spinal cord lesions typically are marked by lower motor neuron (LMN) weakness at the level of the lesion, usually in a nerve root, or by a radicular pattern, with bilateral upper motor neuron (UMN) weakness, including spasticity, hyperreflexia, and positive Babinski signs, occurring below the lesion. Spinal cord lesions that affect all four extremities show no enhanced jaw jerk, which distinguishes them from lesions at higher levels of the neuraxis.

Modified with permission from Feske S. Neurologic history and examination. In: Samuels MA, Feske S, eds. *Office Practice of Neurology*. New York: Churchill Livingstone; 1996.

Nerve Root Lesions in the Upper Extremity

	C5	C6	C7	C8	T1
Sensory Loss	Lateral upper arm and deltoid	Lateral forearm, thumb, and index finger	Central forearm, dorsal and volar sides	Medial forearm, little finger	Axilla and medial upper arm
Pain/Paresthesia	Same as above, rarely below elbow	Same as above, and especially index finger	Same as above, and especially middle finger	Same as above, especially little finger	Same as above, especially axilla
Weakness	Supraspinatus Infraspinatus Deltoid Rhomboids Biceps Brachioradialis	Pronator teres Supinator Biceps Brachioradialis	Triceps Wrist extensors Finger extensors Pronator teres Wrist flexors	Finger flexors Wrist flexors Abductor pollicis brevis Extensor indicis proprius	Intrinsic hand muscles Abductor pollicis brevis
Reflex Loss	Biceps, Brachioradialis	Brachioradialis, Biceps	Triceps	Finger jerks	None

Cervical radiculopathy is a common neurological problem. Because dermatomal and myotomal territories overlap, it is often difficult to localize neurological deficits to a single nerve root. Two principles may help: Paresthesia, when present, localizes more accurately than pain; and findings of weakness in the upper extremity may localize better than sensory findings, due to greater overlap of sensory territories. The most common causes of cervical radiculopathy vary according to location: C5 radiculopathy is often due to cervical spondylosis or upper brachial plexus trauma, C6 and C7 radiculopathy is usually caused by cervical spondylosis or disk protrusion, C8 and T1 lesions can be caused by thoracic outlet syndrome or Pancoast tumor. In the latter case, an ipsilateral Horner's syndrome often accompanies the nerve root findings.

Stewart (2000); Preston and Shapiro (1998).

Nerve Root Lesions in the Lower Extremity

	L2	L3	L4	L5	S1
Sensory Loss	Anterior and lateral thigh	Anterior and medial thigh	Medial leg to medial ankle	Anterior and lateral leg to dorsum of foot and big toe	Sole and lateral border of foot
Pain/Paresthesia	Same as above	Same as above, especially around knee	Same as above	Same as above	Same as above, and especially back of thigh and calf
Weakness	Psoas	Psoas Rectus femoris Vastus medialis/ lateralis Adductors	Tibialis anterior Rectus femoris Vastus medialis/ lateralis Adductors	Tibialis anterior Toe extensors	Gastrocnemius Toe flexors
Reflex Loss	None	Knee	Knee	None	Ankle jerk

Similar principles apply to lumbar/sacral radiculopathy as for cervical radiculopathy (see *Nerve Root Lesions in the Upper Extremity*). However, in the lower extremity, sensory findings may localize better than weakness, due to greater overlap of motor territories. Disk protrusion is a common cause of L5 and S1 radiculopathy; lesions of the L2–L4 roots are more commonly due to neoplasm, such as neurofibroma, meningioma, or metastasis.

Stewart (2000); Preston and Shapiro (1998).

Root vs. Nerve Lesions in the Extremities

Root vs. Nerve	Features in Common	Distinguishing Features	
		C7	Radial
C7 vs. Radial	Weakness of triceps and wrist extensors	Weakness of wrist flexors	Weakness of brachioradialis
	Loss of triceps jerk	Sensory changes over middle finger	Sensory changes, if any, over thumb and index finger
		C8	Median
C8 vs. Median	Weakness of flexor digitorum super-ficialis to all digits	Weakness of flexor digitorum pro-fundus in ring and little fingers	No weakness of flexor digitorum profundus in ring and little fingers
	Pain may spread up forearm to elbow	Sensory loss includes little finger, heel of hand, and medial forearm	Sensory loss con-fined to first three digits and heel of hand below the wrist
		T1	Ulnar
T1 vs. Ulnar	Weakness of small muscles of hand	Weakness of ab-ductor pollicis brevis	Weakness of flexor carpi ulnaris
	Minimal sensory loss	Pain in shoulder and axilla	Pain in ring and little fingers, sometimes spreading to elbow
		L5	Common Peroneal
L5 vs. Common Peroneal	Weakness of foot dorsiflexion	Little weakness of foot eversion	Marked weakness of foot eversion
		May have sensory change in lateral buttock	Sensory change confined to be-low the knee

Lesions of certain roots and nerves subserving the extremities can resemble each other. Knowledge of specific differences in their innervation patterns allows one to differentiate between root and nerve etiology.

Stewart (2000).

Coma

Etiology	Percent of Total
Infectious, metabolic, or diffuse causes	65
Drug intoxication	30
Mixed or nonspecific metabolic	10
Hepatic encephalopathy	3
Hypoglycemia	3
Encephalitis	3
Subarachnoid bleed	3
Endocrine (including diabetes)	2
Other causes	11
Supratentorial lesions	20
Hemorrhage	15
Intracerebral	9
Subdural	5
Epidural	1
Stroke	2
Tumor	1
Abscess	1
Infratentorial lesions	13
Brainstem stroke	8
Pontine bleed	2
Cerebellar bleed	1
Psychiatric disorders	2
Conversion disorder	1
Catatonia	<1
Depression	<1

These statistics are derived from a study of 500 inpatients for whom the initial diagnosis was unclear and thus excludes obvious causes of coma such as trauma or other preestablished diagnoses.

Plum and Posner (1982).

Episodic Loss of Consciousness

Cause	Clinical Features
Syncopal causes	
Hypotension	The most common cause of syncope is so-called vaso-vagal syncope, occurring often in young persons in response to emotional stimuli. Onset is usually gradual, with lightheadedness, graying of vision, and sympathetic signs. Other causes of hypotension include hypovolemia or autonomic dysfunction.
Cardiac arrhythmia	Rapid onset, occasionally with palpitations. Etiologies include AV and SA block and supraventricular and ventricular tachyarrhythmias. Long QT syndrome is a rare, inherited cause of tachyarrhythmia seen in the young.
Decreased cardiac output	Due to valvular obstruction, ventricular dysfunction, or pulmonary embolism.
Cerebrovascular ischemia	Lightheadedness and bilateral motor or sensory deficits due to ischemia in either carotid or vertebrobasilar circulation. The latter may occur in the setting of neck extension or head turning but probably is overdiagnosed as a cause of fainting.
Epileptic causes	
Generalized tonic-clonic seizures	Loss of consciousness with prolonged rhythmic jerking of the extremities (not to be confused with brief jerks that can occur with loss of posture in syncope).
Complex partial seizures	May not be associated with convulsions but usually with a postictal state. Often has a prodrome (aura) of unusual sensory or emotional sensations.
Absence seizures	Brief loss of consciousness without loss of posture or postictal state. Associated with childhood epilepsy syndromes and is rare in adults (often confused with complex partial seizures).
Psychogenic seizures (pseudoseizures)	Paroxysmal spells that appear similar to seizures but are not associated with EEG changes. Often difficult to diagnose without EEG monitoring. See *Features of Psychogenic Seizures (Pseudoseizures)* in Chapter 5.
Other causes	
Breath holding	Loss of consciousness in young children associated with cyanosis or pallor, usually triggered by an emotional or painful stimulus.
Increased intracranial pressure	Due to obstruction of cerebrospinal fluid circulation, such as colloid cyst of the third ventricle.

SA: sinoatrial; AV: atrioventricular.

Bruni (1996).

Syncope vs. Seizure

Clinical Feature	Syncope	Seizure
Relation to posture	Common	No
Skin changes	Pale color, sweaty	Normal color or cyanosis
Aura or warning signs	Lightheadedness, dimmed vision, palpitations	Paresthesias, flashing lights; olfactory, visceral, or emotional symptoms (CP seizures); or none
Duration of aura or warning symptoms	Long	Usually brief, except with CP seizures
Convulsion	Rare	Common
Injury	Rare	Common
Urinary incontinence, tongue biting	Rare	Common
Postevent confusion	Rare	Common
Cardiovascular signs	Common (in cardiac syncope)	No
Abnormal EEG	Rare	Common

CP: complex partial.

The distinction between syncope and seizure is best made on the basis of a careful history. A description of the signs and symptoms preceding the attack (with sympathetic signs and symptoms favoring syncope) and those following the attack (postevent confusion or headache lasting more than several minutes favors seizure) usually make the diagnosis. Additional studies, such as EEG or Holter monitoring, may be necessary for confirmation.

Bruni (1996).

Acute Confusion

Cause	Common Precipitants
Toxins	Alcohol
	Street drugs: amphetamines, PCP
	Anticholinergic medications: TCAs, cogentin, scopolamine
	Other medications: benzodiazepines, AEDs, theophylline
Infection	Urinary tract
	Lung
	CNS: meningitis, encephalitis, meningeal carcinomatosis
Electrolyte disorder	Hyper- or hypoglycemia due to diabetes mellitus
	Hyper- or hyponatremia
	Hypercalcemia due to bone malignancy
	Hepatic or uremic dysfunction
Seizure	History of epilepsy
	Alcohol withdrawal
	CNS infection or mass
Head injury	Often occult and in setting of alcohol abuse
CNS lesion	Stroke
	Brain tumor, especially right hemisphere
	Migraine
Nutritional deficiency	Thiamine
	B_{12}
	B_6
Psychiatric	Exacerbation of bipolar or thought disorder
	Sleep deprivation
	ICU psychosis

PCP: phencyclidine; TCAs: tricyclic antidepressants; AEDs: antiepileptic drugs.

Confusion is the loss of cognitive capabilities marked by prominent inattentiveness. The most common causes, in approximate order of frequency, are listed here. In the young, the most common cause is toxic; in the elderly, or those with baseline diminished cognitive functions, the most common cause is an infection, usually systemic. However, a broad initial workup of the acutely confused patient requires toxic screen, CBC and serum panel, lumbar puncture, and head imaging. The distinctive triad of confusion, gait instability, and abnormal eye movements should be recognized as Wernicke's syndrome and urgently treated with thiamine.

Ronthal (1996); Purdie, Honigman, and Rosen (1981).

Delirium vs. Psychosis

Feature	Delirium	Psychosis
Onset	Sudden	Sudden
Course	Fluctuating	Stable
Consciousness	Reduced	Clear
Cognition	Globally disordered due to inattention	May be selectively impaired
Hallucinations	Visual or visual and auditory	Auditory
Involuntary movements	Asterixis or tremor	Usually absent
Physical illness or drug toxicity	Usually present	Usually absent

Delirium is a state of agitated confusion, marked by significant inattention, and usually due to drug toxicity or systemic illness. An acute exacerbation of a psychotic disorder can be differentiated from delirium by the findings of a relatively preserved level of consciousness and relatively constant clinical course.

Reprinted with permission from Sumner AD, Simons RJ. Delirium in the elderly. *Cleve Clin J Med.* 1994.

Common Cognitive Dysfunction Syndromes (by deficit on mental status testing)

Syndrome	Attention	Mood	Language	Visual Processing	Memory	Executive Functions	Anatomic Site
Acute confusion	●		○	○	○		Frontal networks
Depression	○	●	○	○	○	○	Projection systems
Aphasia			●				Left hemisphere
Hemispatial neglect	○	○		●			Right hemisphere
Balint syndrome				●			Bilateral parietooccipital
Alzheimer's disease	○	○	○	○	●		Limbic system
Schizophrenia	●	○				●	Frontal networks

● domain most affected; ○ domain may be affected. *Executive functions* include social skills, judgment, and insight.

Modified with permission from Weintraub S. Examining mental state. In: Samuels MA, Feske S, eds. *Office Practice of Neurology*. New York: Churchill Livingstone; 1996:705.

Acute Monocular Vision Loss

Disease	Clinical Features
Central retinal artery occlusion	Sudden, painless loss of entire visual field Deficit maximal at onset Little or no afferent pupillary defect Infarct visualizable on dilated fundoscopy
Transient monocular blindness (amaurosis fugax)	Sudden, usually partial, loss of vision lasting minutes to hours Visual field defect usually "altitudinal"; that is, defect boundary is horizontal, with onset perceived as "a curtain falling down" Normal findings on fundoscopy Usually due to embolism, especially in elderly
Anterior ischemic optic neuropathy	Sudden painless central or paracentral vision loss Afferent pupillary defect and loss of color saturation (dyschromotopsia) Risk factors: atherosclerosis, HTN, DM Slow progression may represent compressive optic neuropathy from a neoplastic source and should be evaluated with head imaging
Optic neuritis	Painful central or paracentral vision loss Onset more gradual than ischemic optic neuropathy, usually over several days Afferent pupillary defect and loss of color saturation (dyschromotopsia) Demyelinative lesion of optic nerve, which recovers over weeks to months Evidence for other CNS demyelinative lesions diagnostic of multiple sclerosis should be evaluated with head MRI
Infectious causes	Common cause of visual loss in immunocompromised due to retinopathy (e.g., cytomegalovirus)

Monocular visual loss can be divided roughly into retinal and optic nerve causes. The latter are distinguished by the presence of a relative afferent pupillary defect and a disproportionate loss of color vision (red desaturation). With visual loss in the elderly, giant cell arteritis (temporal arteritis) always should be ruled out. Angle-closure glaucoma should be considered in cases of intermittent monocular vision loss.

Pless and Samiy (1999); Lessell (1978).

Binocular Vision Loss

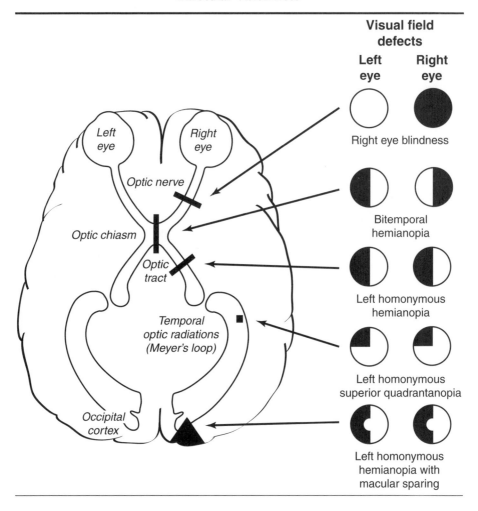

Lesions of the optic pathways produce characteristic patterns of visual field loss. As a rule, prechiasmal lesions produce monocular visual loss. Chiasmal lesions produce bitemporal hemianopia. Retrochiasmal lesions yield homonymous hemianopias with varying degrees of congruence (equal extent of visual field loss in both eyes); lesions that are relatively anterior in the optic radiations tend to produce less congruent field defects. Ischemic lesions of the occipital cortex tend to produce hemianopias with macular sparing, owing to the dual vascular supply of the occipital pole. Superior quadrantanopia is a common sequela to temporal lobectomy for intractable epilepsy.

Tomsak (2000).

Anisocoria

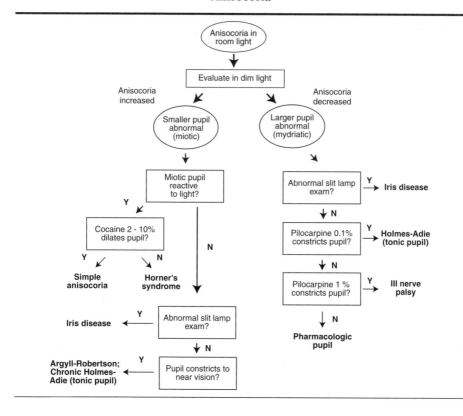

Several causes of anisocoria, or differing pupil sizes between the two eyes, appear most frequently. Simple anisocoria occurs in up to 15% of the population, but the presence of miosis, even without ptosis, should always suggest Horner's syndrome. Topical cocaine administration fails to dilate the sympathetically denervated Horner's pupil, distinguishing the two syndromes. Mydriasis and ptosis in the same eye points to a partial lesion of the III nerve, warranting neuroimaging.

An occasional cause of in-hospital neurologic consultation is unilateral nonreactive mydriasis or "blown pupil." The concern is brainstem herniation, but in the awake patient, the cause is usually accidental application of cholinergic antagonists to the affected eye: eye drops instilled during a previous ophthalmologic consultation, accidental transfer of scopolamine from a transdermal patch on the neck to the eye, or accidental contact with bronchodilator drugs. Failure of the pupils to constrict with pilocarpine drops is confirmatory.

Light-near dissociation, or failure of the eye(s) to constrict to light while still appropriately constricting to near gaze, is seen in Argyll-Robertson pupils; this is a rare entity owing to the near eradication of neurosyphilis, its main cause. The Holmes-Adie pupil is more frequently seen, usually in women, and can progress from a unilateral to a bilateral condition. The mydriasis in Holmes-Adie is due to parasympathetic denervation, and responds to dilute pilocarpine drops.

Cox and Daroff (2000).

19

Diplopia

Cranial Nerve Affected	Normal Eye	Affected Eye	Gaze
III Produces ptosis in the affected eye, which is "down and out" and unable to adduct. Note that here the pupil is dilated, as would be seen with a compressive lesion.			←
			→
IV Causes a subtle vertical diplopia, especially for down gaze. In primary gaze position, the main deficit is a loss of intorsion in the affected eye, for which the patient compensates by tilting the head.			Primary position
			Primary with head tilt
VI The affected eye cannot move laterally to the affected side.			←
			→

Binocular diplopia is caused by a mismatch in eye position in one or more directions of eye movement. There are many causes of eye movement weakness (see *Acute Ophthalmoparesis*), but some of the most common are due to lesions of cranial nerves III, IV, and VI.

Pless and Samiy (1999).

Acute Ophthalmoparesis

Cause	Clinical Features
CNS causes	
Brainstem stroke or mass	Unilateral ophthalmoparesis with contralateral long-tract signs, such as pyramidal weakness
Wernicke's syndrome	Eye movement abnormalities range from nystagmus to bilateral VI weakness and conjugate gaze palsy, to complete ophthalmoplegia, along with gait ataxia and mental status changes in the setting of chronic alcoholism
Cranial nerve causes	
Trauma	IV, VI most affected
Infarction	Painful and pupil sparing, often in setting of DM
Infection or inflammation	Associated with meningitis, Lyme, or sarcoid
Aneurysm of posterior communicating artery	Causes a palsy of III, affecting the pupil (dilated)
Cavernous sinus syndrome	Carotid aneurysm, thrombosis, or infection in cavernous sinus affecting a combination of III, IV, VI, and V_1 or V_2
Superior orbital fissure syndrome	Similar to cavernous sinus syndrome but V_2 is spared
Increased intracranial pressure	VI first affected; III affected with brainstem herniation
Guillain-Barré syndrome (Miller Fisher syndrome)	Bilateral ophthalmoparesis, associated with ataxia, usually in a child
Neuromuscular junction causes	
Myasthenia gravis	Fatigable weakness of eye movements
Botulism	Bilateral, with associated generalized weakness and anticholinergic symptoms: dilated pupils, dry mouth
Ocular muscle causes	
Thyroid disease	Proptosis associated with hyper- or hypothyroidism

Weakness in eye movements causes binocular diplopia and usually is due to a process that affects a single cranial nerve. By far the most common cause in adults is cranial nerve infarction, after affecting the III nerve in the setting of diabetes. III nerve infarction generally does not affect the pupillary innervation, whereas an extrinsic mass lesion, such as a circle of Willis aneurysm, will. In children, head trauma is a common cause of ophthalmoparesis.

Liu (1996).

Gaze Paresis

Cause	Clinical Features
Wernicke's syndrome	Eye movement abnormalities range from nystagmus to bilateral VI weakness and conjugate gaze palsy, to complete ophthalmoplegia, along with gait ataxia and mental status changes in the setting of chronic alcoholism.
Cerebral infarction	Frontal lobe lesions may cause a transient gaze palsy to the contralateral side. Note that the "eyes look at the lesion" in cerebral gaze palsy, whereas in pontine lesions, such as the one-and-a-half syndrome, the gaze palsy is ipsilateral ("wrong-way eyes").
Internuclear ophthalmoplegia (INO)	A lesion of the pontine medial longitudinal fasciculus (MLF), usually demyelinating, causes ipsilateral loss of adduction and contralateral nystagmus with horizontal gaze to the contralateral side. Loss of adduction in both eyes usually is a sign of bilateral INO and is virtually diagnostic of multiple sclerosis.
One-and-a-half syndrome	Lesion of the pontine paramedian reticular formation and neighboring MLF causes loss of all horizontal movement in the ipsilateral eye with preservation of only abduction in the contralateral eye. May be associated with a contralateral hemiparesis.
Parinaud's syndrome	Vertical gaze paresis (upgaze > downgaze), lid retraction, and convergence-retraction nystagmus due to a pineal tumor or hydrocephalus.
Progressive supranuclear palsy	A degenerative disease causing vertical gaze paresis (downgaze > upgaze), dementia, and gait instability.

Gaze paresis is the failure of voluntary *conjugate* eye movements. Lesions affecting conjugate gaze usually are supranuclear; that is, above the level of the III, IV, and VI cranial nerve nuclei. Supranuclear lesions affect voluntary conjugate gaze, but reflex gaze movements, such as those elicited by the doll's head maneuver, will be intact.

Liu (1996).

Abnormal Eye Movements

Movement	Description	Cause
End-gaze nystagmus	Jerking movements with extreme lateral gaze, with fast phase in direction of gaze	Alcohol Anticonvulsants Sedative drugs
Vestibular nystagmus	Peripheral causes: jerking movements with a latency to onset, decay within 1 min, and habituation with repetition	Peripheral: labyrinthitis, vestibular neuronitis, benign positional vertigo, Ménière's disease
	Central causes: no latency, no decay with time, and no habituation	Central: VIII neuropathy, cerebellopontine angle tumor, multiple sclerosis
Upbeat nystagmus	Upward jerking movements when the eyes are in primary gaze position	Structural lesion of brainstem at pontomedullary or pontomesencephalic junctions
Downbeat nystagmus	Downward jerking movements when the eyes are in primary gaze position	Structural lesion at the craniocervical junction, such as Chiari malformation or foramen magnum tumor
Ocular dysmetria	Overshoot or undershoot of a target while visually tracking an object	Cerebellar dysfunction (e.g., vermal atrophy)
Opsoclonus	Chaotic eye saccades in all directions, made worse by attempts to fixate	Viral encephalitis, toxins, and as paraneoplastic sequela (in children, neuroblastoma; in adults, paraneoplastic cerebellar degeneration)
Convergence-retraction nystagmus	Not true nystagmus but an unusual eye movement seen in Parinaud's syndrome: rapid horizontal eye movements with retraction of the globes triggered by attempted upgaze	Lesion of dorsal midbrain, caused by hydrocephalus or pineal region tumor (see *Gaze Paresis*)

Lavin (1996).

Facial Nerve Palsy

Cause	Clinical Features
Bell's palsy	The term given to idiopathic peripheral facial palsy, marked by the subacute onset (1–2 days) of facial weakness that involves the forehead and orbicularis muscles, with variable loss of taste, lacrimation, salivation, and the acoustic reflex (ability to damp out loud sounds at the tympanum). Increasing evidence implicates herpes simplex virus type 1 as the underlying etiology, but Lyme disease also should be suspected in endemic areas.
Ramsay Hunt syndrome	Facial palsy and external ear pain, with the presence of herpes zoster vesicles in the auditory canal and pinna. Due to an outbreak of varicella zoster virus within the sensory afferents of VII. Treated with oral acyclovir or equivalent, unless CNS involvement is apparent, requiring IV therapy.
Trauma	Traumatic facial nerve injuries usually result from a blunt impact to the temporal bone. Consultation is necessary to determine the need for surgical exploration.
Middle ear infection	Infection, usually beginning as otitis media, is a relatively infrequent cause of facial paralysis in the antibiotic era but still is occasionally seen in children and immunocompromised adults. Usually presents as mastoid pain persisting after the acute infection has resolved. Surgical intervention usually is necessary.
Neoplasm	Rarely the VII nerve is compressed in the cerebellopontine angle by a vestibular schwannoma (VIII nerve or acoustic neuroma) or by a schwannoma of VII itself, but more frequently, damage to VII follows surgery for an VIII nerve tumor.

Bauer and Coker (1996).

Bilateral Facial Nerve Palsy

Cause	Percent of Total
Benign	51
Bilateral Bell's palsy	23
Guillain-Barré syndrome	12
Multiple cranial neuropathy	7
Brainstem encephalitis, Miller Fisher syndrome, pseudotumor cerebri	<5 each
Neoplastic	21
Meningeal carcinomatosis	9
Prepontine neoplasms	7
Pontine glioma	<5
Infectious	12
Syphilis, Hansen's disease, cryptococcal meningitis/AIDS, TB meningitis	<5 each
Other	16
Diabetes, sarcoidosis, head trauma, SLE, pontine hemorrhage	<5 each

Facial weakness due to a lesion of the VII nerve most frequently is due to idiopathic Bell's palsy. In about 7% of cases of Bell's palsy, facial weakness is recurrent. Even less frequently seen is simultaneous bilateral VII nerve palsy, occurring less than 1% as often as unilateral VII palsy. The most frequent cause of bilateral VII palsy remains idiopathic, but its appearance should raise questions about other, more ominous conditions, such as meningitis or meningeal carcinomatosis, which may deserve further workup. In addition, Lyme disease may be a frequent cause of "idiopathic" Bell's palsy and should be suspected in endemic areas.

Modified with permission from Keane JR. Bilateral seventh nerve palsy: analysis of 43 cases and review of the literature. *Neurology.* 1994;44:1198–1202.

Halperin and Golightly (1992).

Hearing Loss

Cause	Examples	Comments
Idiopathic	Presbycusis	Most common cause of hearing loss, particularly in elderly; high frequencies most affected
	Ménière's disease	Low-frequency hearing loss and tinnitus with episodes of vertigo, also usually in elderly
Infectious	Labyrinthitis	Viral infection of inner ear causing severe vertigo and hearing loss
	Meningitis	VIII nerve damage due to basilar exudates
Trauma	Tympanic membrane perforation; temporal bone fracture	Trauma can cause conductive or sensorineural hearing loss; hemotympanum or Battle's sign suggests temporal fracture
Noise	Occupational exposure; explosion	Hearing loss centered around 4,000 Hz
Neoplasm	Vestibular schwannoma (acoustic neuroma)	Auditory discrimination deficit is out of proportion to hearing loss; may have accompanying VII nerve palsy
Drugs	Aminoglycosides; cis-platinum; salicylates	Tinnitus and hearing loss due to salicylates (aspirin) is reversible; other causes are irreversible
Autoimmune	Cogan's syndrome; temporal arteritis; SLE	Rapidly progressive hearing loss in setting of autoimmune disease; treatment requires steroids or other immunosuppressants
Pontine lesions	Stroke; multiple sclerosis	More likely to cause deficits in auditory discrimination than frank hearing loss

Vernick (1996); Hughes et al. (1996).

Dizziness

Symptom	Distinguishing Features	Causes
Vertigo	Illusion of motion (usually spinning) Nausea or vomiting Disequilibrium ± Hearing loss/tinnitus	VIII nerve causes: Motion sickness Vestibular neuronitis Benign positional vertigo Ménière's disease CNS causes: Brainstem ischemia Posterior fossa mass Basilar migraine Multiple sclerosis
Syncope or presyncope	Faint, lightheaded feeling Diaphoresis, pale color Graying or loss of vision May be triggered by emotional stimulus or environment (heat)	Cardiac causes: Vasovagal Arrhythmia Left ventricular dysfunction Carotid sinus hypersensitivity Orthostatic causes: Volume depletion Drug-induced Autonomic insufficiency
Disequilibrium	Sense of imbalance without vertigo ± Proprioceptive deficit ± Cerebellar dysfunction ± Extrapyramidal motor dysfunction	Peripheral neuropathy Subacute combined degeneration Tabes dorsalis Posterior fossa mass or infarction Visual loss Extrapyramidal disease (e.g., Parkinson's)
Ill-defined	Poorly described dizziness with no features of other categories	Hyperventilation Depression or anxiety

Dizziness is a term used by patients to describe a wide variety of symptoms, including vertigo, presyncope, and disequilibrium. The differential diagnosis of dizziness can be approached by first determining which of the preceding four categories best fits the associated signs and symptoms.

Weiss (1995).

Vertigo

Cause	Distinguishing Features
Vestibular neuronitis; viral labyrinthitis	Sudden onset of prolonged vertigo, nausea or vomiting ± Tinnitus with hearing intact No focal neurologic signs Often affects young persons
Benign positional vertigo	Brief episodes of vertigo prompted by change in position (often rolling over in bed) Provocative maneuver shows nystagmus of short duration, with a latent period, and fatigable
Posttraumatic vertigo	Persistent or brief episodes of vertigo precipitated by head movement History of head trauma
Ménière's disease	Episodic severe vertigo Feeling of fullness in ear and tinnitus Hearing loss, often progressive
Brainstem ischemia	Mild to moderate vertigo Accompanying brainstem signs (e.g., ataxia, hemiparesis, sensory loss, diplopia) Rare hearing loss Provocative maneuver shows nystagmus of long duration, with no latent period, and not fatigable
Posterior fossa mass or infarction	Acute, severe vertigo (infarction) or slowly progressive vertigo (mass) Limb ataxia ipsilateral to lesion ± Brainstem signs (hemiparesis, sensory loss) ± Intractable nausea or vomiting and decreased level of consciousness (infarction with edema or hemorrhage)
Basilar migraine	Recurrent attacks of vertigo followed by severe headache Accompanying visual deficits, sensory symptoms (numbness and tingling in hands, feet, and lips) Onset usually in childhood

Weiss (1995).

Dysarthria

Dysarthria Type	Speech Features	Typical Causes
Lower motor neuron	Slurred, indistinct speech: loss of *r* sounds with early weakness; later loss of labial *m, b, p* sounds and lingual *l* and *t* sounds May be associated with dysphagia, facial weakness, or generalized muscular weakness	Lower cranial nerve palsies (VII, X, XII) Neuromuscular disease (Guillain-Barré, myasthenia gravis)
Upper motor neuron	Strained, strangled speech, produced at a slow rate May be associated with signs of pseudobulbar palsy: dysphagia, increased jaw jerk, increased "emotional" facial expression reflexes	Stroke Multiple sclerosis Amyotrophic lateral sclerosis
Rigid	Hypophonic, monotonous speech that is slurred and speeded up so that words run together	Hypokinetic extrapyramidal movement disorders such as Parkinson's disease
Hyperkinetic	Loud speech that is erratically stressed; speech may be arrested by superimposed abnormal movements	Hyperkinetic movement disorders such as Huntington's chorea
Ataxic	Slow, slurred speech that is monotonous and has long breaks between syllables (scanning)	Acute or chronic cerebellar disease
Stuttering	Interruption of speech by repetition or arrest on single syllables or sounds	Developmental condition or may be a transient stage of recovery from nonfluent aphasia

Dysarthria, or abnormal articulation of speech, usually occurs in the setting of other neurological deficits. The abnormal qualities of speech often reflect the characteristics of the underlying neurological syndrome.

Adams, Victor, and Ropper (1997:489–490).

Acute Generalized Weakness

Cause	Distinguishing Features
Guillain-Barré syndrome (GBS)	Ascending paralysis Little or no sensory loss Areflexia Antecedent viral illness
Tick paralysis	Ascending paralysis in children resembling GBS Due to toxin from *Dermacentor* tick species Removal of tick reverses symptoms
Miller Fisher syndrome	Weakness with marked ataxia, ophthalmoplegia, and areflexia
Myasthenia gravis	Predominantly bulbar weakness Fluctuating course Preservation of reflexes
Botulism	Bulbar weakness followed by descending paralysis Autonomic signs and symptoms: dilated pupils, dry mouth, and constipation
Metabolic or toxic abnormality	
Hypermagnesemia	Obstetric patient being treated for eclampsia or preeclampsia
Hypophosphatemia	Patient undergoing parenteral alimentation
Hypokalemic periodic paralysis	History of episodic weakness
Organophosphate toxicity	Weakness and cholinergic symptoms (diarrhea, vomiting, sweating) due to insecticide exposure
Biological toxins (ciguatera, pufferfish, etc.)	History of marine fish ingestion
Cervical spinal cord lesion	Weakness plus sensory level Bowel and bladder dysfunction Neck pain
Critical illness polyneuropathy	Limb weakness with spared cranial nerves Difficulty weaning from mechanical ventilation History of sepsis or multiorgan failure
Poliomyelitis	Ascending paralysis, usually asymmetric Signs and symptoms of viral meningitis Recent treatment with oral polio vaccine

Pascuzzi and Fleck (1997).

Muscle Weakness

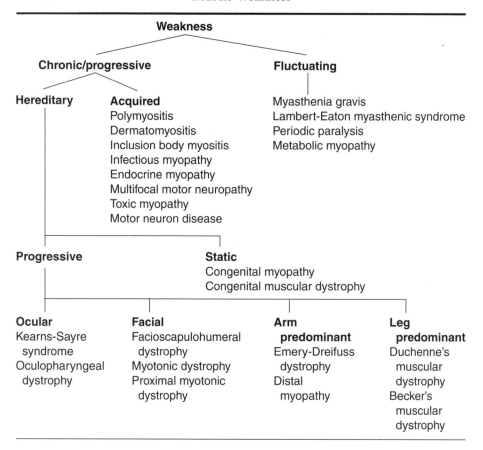

Modified with permission from Cwik VA, Brooke MH. Proximal, distal and generalized weakness. In: Bradley WG, Daroff RB, Fenichel GM, Marsden CD, eds. *Neurology in Clinical Practice.* 2nd ed. Boston: Butterworth-Heinemann; 1996. Differential provided by K. Boonyapisit and H. J. Kaminski.

Muscle Fatigue

Disease	Clinical Features	Molecular Mechanism
Myasthenia gravis	Weakness of ocular, bulbar, neck, and shoulder girdle muscles most prominent; weakness increases during short periods of activity and tends to increase overall over course of day	Autoantibodies to acetylcholine receptor
Lambert-Eaton myasthenic syndrome	Weakness of proximal muscles of extremities and trunk; weakness increases after brief periods of exertion, but may paradoxically decrease during first few muscle contractions	Autoantibodies to presynaptic calcium channels; associated with oat-cell lung carcinoma, as well as other cancers
Myophosphorylase deficiency (McArdle's disease); Phosphofructokinase deficiency	Weakness and pain in the extremities after strenuous exercise; strength may return after a brief rest ("second wind"); myoglobinuria is common; usually diagnosed in adolescence or young adulthood	Defect in glycogenosis due to AR inheritance of enzyme deficiency
Carnitine palmitoyl-transferase deficiency	Attacks of weakness, pain, and muscle cramping during prolonged athletic activity; weakness cannot be reversed by a brief rest; possible severe myoglobinuria leading to renal compromise	Defect in fatty acid metabolism due to AR inheritance of enzyme deficiency
Hypokalemic periodic paralysis	Rapid onset of diffuse weakness that follows strenuous exercise or heavy carbohydrate ingestion; weakness lasts hours to days, then gradually reverses; serum K^+ may drop below 2 mM	AD inheritance of mutation in a subunit of voltage-gated calcium channels
Hyperkalemic periodic paralysis	Brief attacks of diffuse weakness (lasting up to an hour) occurring early or late in the day after exercise; recovery may be speeded by mild exercise; serum K^+ may rise to 5–6 mM	AD inheritance of mutation in a subunit of voltage-gated sodium channels

Abnormal muscle fatigue is most frequently due to myasthenia gravis or its paraneoplastic counterpart, Lambert-Eaton myasthenic syndrome. These diseases usually present in the middle-aged or elderly. A few inherited syndromes can cause dramatic fatiguable weakness and usually are diagnosed by young adulthood.

Adams, Victor, and Ropper (1997:1432–1448, 1476–1488).

Proximal Weakness

Feature	Neuronopathy	Myopathy	Myasthenia
Tendon reflexes	Absent	Depressed or absent	Normal
EMG	Fasciculations; fibrillations; high-amplitude, polyphasic motor units	Brief, small-amplitude, polyphasic motor units	Normal
Nerve conduction	Normal or mildly slow	Normal	Abnormal repetitive stimulation
CK level	Normal or mildly high	High (inflammatory) Normal (metabolic)	Normal
Muscle biopsy	Group atrophy; group typing	Fiber necrosis, fatty replacement; excessive collagen	Normal

Progressive proximal weakness most often is due to a myopathic disease process, such as muscular dystrophy in the young or inflammatory muscle disease in the elderly. Other causes that should be considered include myasthenia (with a history of fatigable weakness) or a neuronopathy such as spinal muscular atrophy (with a family history). Electrodiagnostic testing provides a means for differentiating among these three broad categories of disease.

Modified with permission from Fenichel GM. *Clinical Pediatric Neurology*. Philadelphia: W.B. Saunders Co.; 1997:179.

Hemiparesis

Anatomic Site	Distinguishing Features
Cerebral cortex	Loss of higher cognitive functions Loss of discriminative sensation Face and arm may be more affected than leg
Cerebral white matter or internal capsule	Loss of higher cognitive functions Loss of discriminative sensation Face, arm, and leg may be equally affected
Brainstem	Cranial nerve dysfunction ipsilateral to lesion ("crossed" to the side of limb weakness)
Cervical spinal cord	Limb weakness ipsilateral to lesion Ipsilateral loss of touch and position sense Contralateral loss of pain and temperature sensation No facial weakness

Hemiparesis is the distinctive pattern of a corticospinal tract lesion, manifest by limb weakness on one side of the body, usually with lower face weakness as well. Established corticospinal tract weakness is accompanied by the signs of upper motor neuron pathology: pyramidal distribution weakness (upper limb extensors and lower limb flexors disproportionately affected), spasticity, and hyperreflexia. The likely pathology underlying hemiparesis depends on the clinical course of weakness: Stroke is the predominant cause of acute hemiparesis; mass lesions such as tumor or abscess cause progressive hemiparesis; and demyelinating disease (or, rarely, migraine) is a common cause of remitting or fluctuating hemiparesis.

Adams, Victor, and Ropper (1997:59–60).

Paraparesis

Acute paraparesis in children and adults	Spinal cord trauma
	Vertebral disk protrusion
	Epidural abscess
	Anterior spinal artery occlusion
	Aortic dissection
	Guillain-Barré syndrome
	Transverse myelitis
	Poliomyelitis
Chronic paraparesis in children	Cerebral palsy
	Congenital spinal cord malformation
	Muscular dystrophy
	Friedreich's ataxia
	Hereditary motor and sensory neuropathy
Chronic paraparesis in adults	Multiple sclerosis
	Spinal cord tumor
	Syringomyelia
	Subacute combined degeneration (B_{12} deficiency)
	HIV myelopathy
	Tropical spastic paraparesis
	Motor neuron disease
	Peripheral neuropathy
	Cerebral parasagittal mass lesion (rare)

Acute paralysis of both lower extremities usually points to the spinal cord as the affected site, which usually is accompanied by the findings of a sensory level and bowel or bladder dysfunction. Guillain-Barré syndrome in its early stages can be confused for spinal cord disease but usually does not present with sphincter dysfunction. Acute paraparesis with back pain should prompt investigation of a structural lesion such as disk, epidural abscess, or aortic dissection with disruption of segmental spinal arteries. Chronic, progressive paraparesis can be caused by spinal cord, peripheral nerve, or muscle disease, and so requires a broader diagnostic approach.

Adams, Victor, and Ropper (1997:60–61).

Headache

Disorder	Clinical Features
Migraine with aura (classic migraine)	Unilateral, pulsating pain of moderate to severe intensity, lasting 4–72 hr Nausea, vomiting, photo- or phonophobia Aura usually of visual phenomena in both visual fields that start centrally and move peripherally: zig-zag bright white lines (fortifications) or focal area of lost vision (scotoma) Sensory aura consists of tingling and numbness, usually starting at the hand and spreading to the mouth over minutes Motor weakness as a migrainous aura is infrequent and only rarely expressed as true paresis Female predominance
Migraine without aura (common migraine)	Pain and associated nausea, vomiting, photo- and phonophobia, and female predominance, which is similar to migraine with aura Absence of aura may make this syndrome more difficult to distinguish from tension headache
Tension headache	Nonpulsating pain (pressure) of mild to moderate intensity Bilateral location No nausea or vomiting but possible photo- or phonophobia If occurs at least 15 days per month over 6 months, may be "chronic tension headache"
Cluster headache	Severe unilateral pain, usually in an orbital or temporal location, lasting 15–180 min if untreated Attacks occur in clusters lasting days to weeks, separated by long attack-free intervals Accompanied by conjunctival injection, rhinorrhea, tearing, and/or nasal congestion on the same side as the pain Male predominance

Olesen (1993); Solomon (1997).

Malignant Causes of Headache

Etiology	Distinguishing Features
Intracranial mass	Symptoms of increased intracranial pressure (headache worse in the morning, worse with cough, or progressively worse over days to weeks) Papilledema Focal neurologic deficit New onset seizure
Transient ischemic attack (TIA)	March of symptoms in seconds (vs. minutes in migraine) Symptoms of sensory deficit (vs. positive symptoms in migraine) Recovery of deficit in minutes
Intracranial bleeding	Sudden onset of severe headache; "worst headache of my life" Meningismus, photophobia, altered level of consciousness
Pseudotumor cerebri	Symptoms of increased intracranial pressure (as above) Papilledema Blurred vision or visual field deficits More frequent in young, obese women
Chronic meningitis	Severe and persistent headache Fever Cranial neuropathy
Colloid cyst of III ventricle	Intermittent severe headache sometimes with nausea or vomiting and rapid changes in level of consciousness
Temporal arteritis	Elderly person with systemic symptoms (fatigue, weight loss) Visual loss Elevated sedimentation rate
Subdural hematoma	Elderly person with history of trauma or fall (may be occult)
Low pressure headache	Headache worse with standing and relieved by recumbency History of lumbar puncture, head trauma, or surgery causing CSF leak

A headache syndrome of years' standing virtually always is benign. Rather, new-onset headache deserves the most diagnostic attention, particularly new-onset headache in a middle-aged or elderly person, headache that becomes progressively worse, or the sudden onset of "the worst headache of my life."

Campbell and Sakai (1993).

Risk Factors for Pseudotumor Cerebri

Factor	Percent of Total
Female gender	83
Obesity	62
Hypertension	17
Oral contraceptives	15
Tetracycline	12
Menstrual irregularity	12
Corticosteroids	10
Thyroid hormone therapy	8
Pregnancy	6
Hypervitaminosis A	4
Sarcoidosis	4
Ulcerative colitis	4
Lupus	2

Pseudotumor cerebri (idiopathic intracranial hypertension; IIH) is a syndrome of elevated intracranial pressure with no underlying mass lesion or CSF abnormality. Aside from chronic headache, a significant fraction of patients suffer visual loss from optic neuropathy. IIH predominantly affects young, obese women. These data show accompanying risk factors in a small sample of patients newly diagnosed with IIH. Some risk factors, such as oral contraceptive use and pregnancy, probably are not genuine risks per se but merely associated with women of childbearing age.

Modified with permission from Jones JS, Nevai J, Freeman MP, McNinth DE. Emergency department presentation of idiopathic intracranial hypertension. *Am J Emerg Med.* 1999; 17:517–521.

Radhakrishnan et al. (1994).

Facial Pain

Disease	Clinical Features
Trigeminal neuralgia	Paroxysmal, severe, lancinating pain in the unilateral distribution of V nerve, usually V_2 or V_3 Triggered by sensory stimulation of face, chewing, or speaking No trigeminal sensory or motor deficit Occurs mostly in elderly Responsive to AEDs such as CBZ or PHT or microvascular decompression
Glossopharyngeal neuralgia	Similar to trigeminal neuralgia, with pain affecting the tonsillar bed and auditory canal
Postherpetic neuralgia	Sequela of facial shingles, usually in elderly Steady, severe burning pain Associated sensory loss at site of old vesicular eruption Somewhat responsive to TCAs, SSRIs
Temporomandibular joint (TMJ) pain (Costen's syndrome)	Pain with chewing arising at the TMJ and radiating over the cheek and face May have TMJ tenderness to palpation Due to malocclusion of molars, may be responsive to bite adjustment by dentist
Dental pain	Maxillary or mandibular pain, usually with a throbbing component, worse at night Tooth tenderness
Atypical facial pain	Aching, throbbing pain in teeth Unresponsive to dental procedures, analgesia, or narcotics May respond to SSRIs
Structural lesion of V	Pain usually is steady and often unresponsive to medication Associated sensory loss in V distribution Loss of ipsilateral corneal reflex May have ipsilateral VII or VIII nerve involvement Workup requires neuroimaging

CBZ: carbamazepine; PHT: phenytoin.

Facial pain often has distinctive features that allow rapid recognition of the underlying syndrome. Benign causes of facial pain have no associated cranial nerve dysfunction; the finding of facial numbness always should trigger a careful workup for a structural lesion, such as cerebellopontine mass or nasopharyngeal carcinoma.

Miller (1968).

Back Pain That Is Surgically Treatable

Intervertebral disk herniation

Local pain plus radicular pain and neurologic deficits due to compromise of nerve roots. The most common sites of protrusion are the L5/S1 disk (affecting the S1 root, with pain from the posterior thigh to the lateral foot and little toe and weakness in foot eversion and plantar flexion) and L4/L5 disk (affecting the L5 root, with pain from the posterior thigh to the foot dorsum and great toe and weakness in foot dorsiflexion). Large protrusions may affect multiple lumbar roots, yielding a cauda equina syndrome.

Lumbar stenosis

Spondylotic changes in the spinal canal cause compression of multiple lumbar roots. The patient experiences the gradual onset of pain, numbness, and weakness of the legs that begins with walking and requires a rest period of sitting or lying (hence, flexing the spine) to relieve the symptoms. This "spinal claudication" can be distinguished from peripheral vascular claudication in that the latter's symptoms can be reversed if the patient merely stops walking and remains standing.

Metastatic vertebral disease

Many types of carcinoma will metastasize to the vertebral column, including breast, lung, prostate, and multiple myeloma. These cause destructive lesions of bone, sparing the disk space. The back pain is described as dull, constant, and worse at night and with recumbency. Bone scan may be necessary to visualize vertebral metastasis in its early stages.

Infectious vertebral disease

Staphylococci and tuberculosis, among others, will invade the vertebral column, causing disk space erosion and back pain with local tenderness to percussion. Local pain, tenderness, and fever always should raise concern of spinal epidural abscess, a neurologic emergency that can cause acute spinal cord compression.

Spinal arteriovenous malformation (AVM)

A rare but serious cause of rapidly evolving severe back pain and spinal cord compression due to bleeding. More commonly, spinal AVMs present as the cause of chronic progressive myelopathy. Angiography usually is required to demonstrate their presence.

The causes of back pain that are not surgically amenable are myriad and often poorly defined, such as "low back strain" and "facet syndrome." This list suggests some syndromes where surgical consultation is advised.

Adams, Victor, and Ropper (1997:194–223).

Patterns of Sensory Loss

Pattern	Modalities Affected	Cause/Examples
	Any	Peripheral neuropathy: (see Chapter 9)
	Position sense Vibration sense	Posterior column spinal cord syndrome: B_{12} deficiency, Friedreich's ataxia
	Pain and temperature	Central spinal cord syndrome: Syringomyelia, Intrinsic spinal cord tumor
	Pain and temperature, contralateral to lesion Position, vibration sense, ipsilateral to lesion All modalities, at lesion	Brown-Séquard syndrome: Extrinsic spinal cord tumor, trauma
	All modalities	Complete spinal cord transection: Trauma, transverse myelitis

Duus (1989).

Movement Disorder	Distinguishing Features	Common Causes
Parkinsonism	Akinesia, rigidity, and tremor	Parkinson's disease Drug-induced parkinsonism "Parkinson's-plus" diseases: PSP, MSA
Resting tremor	Resting tremor relieved by posture Resting tremor made worse by posture (rubral tremor)	Parkinson's disease Lesion of red nucleus or cerebellar outflow
Action tremor	Tremor of extremities or head made worse by posture Tremor of extremities made worse by reaching movements	Essential tremor, enhanced physiologic tremor Intention tremor due to cerebellar dysfunction
Myoclonus	Burst of jerky muscle contractions	Multiple causes at all levels of the nervous system
Asterixis	Brief interruptions of muscle tone during sustained posture ("negative myoclonus")	Metabolic causes such as hepatic dysfunction
Chorea	Rapid, jerky, but coordinated involuntary movements	Huntington's disease Sydenham's chorea
Tics	Rapid, nonrhythmic movements under partial voluntary control	Tourette's syndrome Stimulant side effect (e.g., Ritalin in children)
Tardive dyskinesia	Repetitive involuntary movements, usually of mouth	Side effects of neuroleptic medications
Akathisia	Restless movement of extremities	Side effects of neuroleptic medications
Dystonia	Abnormally increased muscle tone in movement or posture	Neuroleptic-induced acute side effect Task-specific dystonia (e.g., writer's cramp) Inherited dystonia syndromes
Athetosis	Slow, snakelike movements that transition between dystonic postures	Same as for dystonia

PSP: progressive supranuclear palsy; MSA: multisystem atrophy.

The initial diagnosis of movement disorders is best done from a distance to appreciate the overall characteristics of the patient's abnormal movements. The differential diagnosis of movement disorders causing "too little movement" is limited mostly to parkinsonism. The disorders that cause "too much movement" are more varied. Their diagnosis begins with a description of what kind of abnormal movement the patient is making. See also *Movement Disorders*, in Chapter 6.

Samuels (1982).

Ataxia

Cause	Age at Onset	Comment
Acute onset		
Migraine	Children	Ataxia followed by headache
Cerebellar stroke or bleeding	Usually adult	Severe headache and vomiting
Subacute onset		
Viral cerebellitis	Child	Usually before 12 yr
Opsoclonus (paraneoplastic)	Usually child	Associated with neuroblastoma
Miller Fisher syndrome	Child, young adult	With ophthalmoparesis
Multiple sclerosis	Young adult	
Paraneoplastic cerebellar degen.	Usually adult	May be associated with anti-Yo
Alcoholic cerebellar degeneration	Adult	Also seen with chronic PHT use
Hydrocephalus	Any	
Posterior fossa mass	Any	
Toxin exposure	Any	Most common cause in children
Foramen magnum compression	Any	Rare in very young or old
Episodic onset		
Inherited metabolic ataxias	<15 yr	Usually apparent in infancy
Dominant periodic ataxias	<20 yr	
Multiple sclerosis	Young adults	
Intermittent hydrocephalus	Any	Colloid cyst of III ventricle, e.g.
Transient ischemic attacks	Adult	Occurs with other brainstem signs
Chronic progressive		
Hypothyroidism	Young children, adults	
Inherited ataxias	Recessive, <15 yr Dominant, <20 yr	See *Inherited Ataxia* in Chapter 7
Idiopathic degenerative ataxias	Usually <30 yr	
Vitamin E deficiency	Adults	Should always been screened in otherwise idiopathic cases
Alcoholic cerebellar degeneration	Adults	May have history of PHT exposure
Paraneoplastic cerebellar degeneration	Adults	May be associated with anti-Yo
Infectious		
Rubella panencephalitis	Child	
Creutzfeldt-Jakob	Adults	
Hydrocephalus	Any	
Foramen magnum compression	Any	Rare in very young or old

PHT: phenytoin.

Modified with permission from Harding AE. Ataxic disorders. In: Bradley WG, Daroff, RB, Fenichel GM, Marsden CD, eds. *Neurology in Clinical Practice.* 2nd ed. Boston: Butterworth-Heinemann; 1996:289–298.

Gait Disorders

Cause	*Percent of Total*	*Clinical Features*
Frontal gait disorder NPH Multiple strokes Binswanger's disease	20	"Magnetic," slow, shuffling gait Dementia and urinary incontinence (NPH) Abnormal head imaging (strokes and Binswanger's disease)

Sensory imbalance
Sensory neuropathy
Multiple sensory
    deficits
	18	Wide-based, unsteady gait; positive Romberg
		    sign
		Loss of distal position sense and other sen-
		    sory modalities
		Abnormal NCS/EMG

Myelopathy Cervical spondylosis Vitamin B_{12} deficiency	16	Stiff, circumducting gait Spasticity and hyperreflexia Cervical spinal cord compression on neck imaging (cervical spondylosis)

Parkinsonism
Parkinson's disease
Drug-induced
    parkinsonism
PSP
	10	Short-stepped gait with decreased arm swing,
		    difficulty turning and initiating gait
		Tremor and rigidity (Parkinson's)
		Predominant loss of balance and axial rigid-
		    ity with loss of vertical eye movements
		    (PSP)

Cerebellar degeneration	8	Wide-based gait Cerebellar atrophy on head imaging May have history of alcohol abuse
Other Brain tumor Subdural hematoma Depression	8	Depends on underlying cause Occult subdural hematoma sometimes seen in elderly
Toxic or metabolic	6	Altered level of consciousness due to uremia, hepatic failure, or medications
Undetermined	14	

NPH: normal pressure hydrocephalus; PSP: progressive supranuclear palsy.

Gait disorders are seen commonly in the elderly and are due to a variety of causes. The statistical data shown here derive from a sample of 50 patients referred to a neurology clinic and exclude nonneurological causes of gait impairment such as joint deformity.

Modifed with permission from Sudarsky L. Geriatrics: Gait disorders in the elderly. *N Engl J Med* 1990;322:44.

Dermatologic Signs of Neurologic Disease

Skin Sign	Neurologic Disease
Petechial rash in a patient with altered mental status	Meningococcal meningitis
Vesicular rash in dermatomal distribution	Herpes zoster
Papular rash on palms and soles, with centripetal spread in a patient with fever and headache	Rocky Mountain spotted fever
Target erythema or migrating erythema	Lyme disease
Generalized maculo-papular rash with patchy erythema in patient taking antiepileptic drugs	AED hypersensitivity
Malar rash and photosensitive rash	Systemic lupus erythematosus
Purplish eyelid rash and photosensitive rash over neck and shoulders	Dermatomyositis
Reticular erythema (livedo reticularis) in a patient with stroke at a young age	Antiphospholipid antibody (Sneddon's syndrome)
Erethymatous facial plaques and subcutaneous nodules, especially in African-American patient	Sarcoidosis
Oral and genital aphthous ulcers in patient with meningoencephalitis	Behçet's disease
Café au lait spots, axillary or inguinal freckles	Neurofibromatosis type I
Hypopigmented macules and facial angiofibromas in a child with mental retardation and seizures	Tuberous sclerosis
Facial nevus involving the forehead and eyelid in a child with focal neurologic deficits	Sturge-Weber syndrome
Hair and eyelash depigmentation in patient with meningoencephalitis	Vogt-Koyanagi-Harada syndrome

Hurko and Provost (1998); Lisowe, Fleck, and Mirowski (1998).

Signs and Symptoms of Conversion Disorder

Feature	Description
Give-way weakness	Strength that suddenly collapses on testing and appears to vary dramatically depending on how much resistance the examiner offers.
Hoover's sign	When testing lower limb paralysis, a hand placed under the strong leg should detect downward pressure during attempted elevation of the weak leg. Failure to detect contralateral hip extensor activation during elevation of the weak leg suggests absence of effort; detection of hip extensor activation in the weak leg while raising the strong leg demonstrates absence of paralysis in those muscles.
Absence of weakness in automatic activities	The patient who demonstrates a paralyzed extremity under direct testing nonetheless may use it normally while adjusting position in bed or hopping onto the examining table
Distractibility	Psychogenic tremor or abnormal gait may improve while the patient is asked to perform another motor task. Psychogenic tremor is particularly hard to maintain while asked to perform another rhythmic activity.
Effortful ataxic gait or "astasia/abasia"	A psychogenic gait in which the patient makes remarkable, effortful gyrations while maintaining balance. Often the base of the gait is quite narrow, giving the appearance of tightrope walking. The patient appears constantly on the verge of falling but usually does not do so unless someone is nearby to catch him or her.
Nonneurologic sensory loss	Sensory loss that ends sharply on anatomic boundaries, such as at the wrist, or at the midline of the trunk and face, violating innervation patterns. Vibration sense that ends sharply at the midline is one such nonneurologic pattern of sensory loss.

The patient who presents with a conversion disorder is a difficult problem in neurological diagnosis. These are some common presentations of signs and symptoms that suggest psychogenic illness. It is important, however, to bear in mind that conversion disorder is a diagnosis of exclusion, and repeated studies have found a high rate of patients initially given this diagnosis who later are found to have organic causes for their symptoms.

Hayes et al. (1999); Hawkes (1997).

Incidence of Neurologic Disease

Disorder	Incidence per 100,000
Herpes zoster	400
Migraine	250
Acute stroke	150
Herniated lumbosacral disk	150
Epilepsy	50
Dementia	50
Polyneuropathy	40
Bell's palsy	25
Parkinsonism	20
Meningitis	15
Encephalitis	15
Metastatic brain tumor	15
Malignant primary brain tumor	5
Multiple sclerosis	3
Motor neuron disease	2
Guillain-Barré syndrome	2
Muscular dystrophy	0.7
Polymyositis	0.5
Hereditary ataxia	0.4
Hereditary motor and sensory neuropathy	0.2
Acute disseminated encephalomyelitis	0.2
Spinal muscular atrophy	0.2
Wilson's disease	0.1
Creutzfeldt-Jakob disease	0.1

Annual incidence rates for all ages in the United States. Multiple sclerosis incidence is for high-risk areas.

Modified with permission Kurtzke JF. The current neurologic burden of illness and injury in the United States. *Neurology.* 1982:32.

REFERENCES

Adams RD, Victor M, Ropper AH. *Principles of Neurology*. New York: McGraw-Hill; 1997.

Bauer CA, Coker NJ. Update on facial nerve disorders. *Otolaryng Clin North Am*. 1996;29:445–454.

Bruni J. Episodic impairment of consciousness. In: Bradley WG, Daroff RB, Fenichel GM, Marsden CD, eds. *Neurology in Clinical Practice*. 2nd ed. Boston: Butterworth-Heinemann; 1996:11–21.

Campbell JK, Sakai F. Migraine: Diagnosis and differential diagnosis. In: Olesen J, Tfelt-Hansen P, Welch KMA, eds. *The Headaches*. New York: Raven Press; 1993:277–281.

Cox TA, Daroff RB. Pupillary and eyelid abnormalities. In: Bradley WG, Daroff RB, Fenichel GM, Marsden CD, eds. *Neurology in Clinical Practice*. 3rd ed. Boston: Butterworth-Heinemann; 2000:229–238.

Cwik VA, Brooke MH. Proximal, distal and generalized weakness. In: Bradley WG, Daroff RB, Fenichel GM, Marsden CD, eds. *Neurology in Clinical Practice*. 2nd ed. Boston: Butterworth-Heinemann; 1996:359–379.

Duus P. *Topical Diagnosis in Neurology*. New York: Thieme Medical Publishers; 1989:50–57.

Fenichel GM. *Clinical Pediatric Neurology*. Philadelphia: W.B. Saunders Co.; 1997:179.

Feske S. Neurologic history and examination. In: Samuels MA, Feske S, eds. *Office Practice of Neurology*. New York: Churchill Livingstone; 1996:2–9.

Halperin JJ, Golightly M. Lyme borreliosis in Bell's palsy. Long Island Neuroborreliosis Collaborative Study Group. *Neurology* 1992;42:1268–1270.

Hanson MR, Sweeney PJ. Disturbances of lower cranial nerves. In: Bradley WG, Daroff RB, Fenichel GM, Marsden CD, eds. *Neurology in Clinical Practice*. 3rd ed. Boston: Butterworth-Heinemann; 2000:271–284.

Harding AE. Ataxic disorders. In: Bradley WG, Daroff RB, Fenichel GM, Marsden CD, eds. *Neurology in Clinical Practice*. 2nd ed. Boston: Butterworth-Heinemann; 1996:289–298.

Harrison MJG. *Neurological Skills*. London: Butterworths; 1987:31–42.

Hawkes CH. Diagnosis of functional neurological disease. *Br J Hosp Med*. 1997;57:373–377.

Hayes MW, Graham S, Heldorf P, de Moore G, Morris JGL. A video review of the diagnosis of psychogenic gait: Appendix and commentary. *Mov Disorders*. 1999;14:914–921.

Hughes GB, Freedman MA, Haberkamp TJ, Guay ME. Sudden sensorineural hearing loss. *Otolaryng Clin North Am*. 1996;29:393-405.

Hurko O, Provost TT. Neurology and the skin. *J Neurol Neurosurg Psych*. 1998;66:417-430.

Jones JS, Nevai J, Freeman MP, McNinch DE. Emergency department presentation of idiopathic intracranial hypertension. *Am J Emerg Med*. 1999;17:517–521.

Keane JR. Bilateral seventh nerve palsy: analysis of 43 cases and review of the literature. *Neurology.* 1994;44:1198–1202.

Kurtzke JF. The current neurologic burden of illness and injury in the United States. *Neurology.* 1982;32:1207–1214.

Lavin PJM. Eye movement disorders and diplopia. In: Bradley WG, Daroff RB, Fenichel GM, Marsden CD, eds. *Neurology in Clinical Practice.* 2nd ed. Boston: Butterworth-Heinemann; 1996:185–207.

Lessell S. Current concepts in ophthalmology: optic neuropathies. *N Engl J Med.* 1978;299:533–536.

Lisowe JA, Fleck JD, Mirowski GW. Pearls in neurodermatology. *Semin Neurol.* 1998;18:243–255.

Liu GT. Disorders of the eyes and eyelids. In: Samuels MA, Feske S, eds. *Office Practice of Neurology.* New York: Churchill Livingstone; 1996: 40–74.

Miller H. Pain in the face. *Brit Med J* 1968; 2:577–580.

Olesen J. Migraine with aura and its subforms. In: Olesen J, Tfelt-Hansen P, Welch KMA, eds. *The Headaches.* New York: Raven Press; 1993:263–275.

Olson WH, Brumback RA, Gascon G, Iyer V. *Handbook of Symptom-Oriented Neurology.* St. Louis: Mosby; 1994:293–340.

Pascuzzi RM, Fleck JD. Acute peripheral neuropathy in adults. Guillain-Barré syndrome and related variants. *Neurol Clin.* 1997;15:529–547.

Pless M, Samiy N. Ophthalmology. In: Samuels MA, ed. *Hospitalist Neurology.* Boston: Butterworth-Heinemann; 1999:475–496.

Plum F, Posner JB. *Diagnosis of Stupor and Coma.* Philadelphia: F.A. Davis; 1982.

Preston DC, Shapiro BE. *Electromyography and Neuromuscular Disorders: Clinical-Electrophysiologic Correlations.* Boston: Butterworth-Heinemann; 1998:413–432.

Purdie FR, Honigman B, Rosen P. Acute organic brain syndrome: a review of 100 cases. *Ann Emerg Med.* 1981;10:455–461.

Radhakrishnan K, Ahlskog JE, Garrity JA, Kurland LT. Idiopathic intracranial hypertension. *Mayo Clin Proc.* 1994;69:169–180.

Ronthal M. Confusional states and metabolic encephalopathy. In: Samuels MA, Feske S, eds. *Office Practice of Neurology.* New York: Churchill Livingstone; 1996:715–718.

Samuels MA. Sorting out movement disorders. *Patient Care.* 1982;16: 16–45.

Solomon S. Diagnosis of primary headache disorders. *Neurol Clin.* 1997; 15:15–26.

Stewart JD. *Focal Peripheral Neuropathies.* Philadelphia: Lippincott Williams & Wilkins; 2000.

Sudarsky L. Geriatrics: Gait disorders in the elderly. *N Engl J Med.* 1990; 322:1441–1446.

Sumner AD, Simons RJ. Delirium in the elderly. *Cleve Clin J Med.* 1994; 61:258–262.

Tomsak RL. Neuro-ophthalmology: Afferent visual system. In: Bradley WG, Daroff RB, Fenichel GM, Marsden CD, eds. *Neurology in Clinical Practice*. 3rd ed. Boston: Butterworth-Heinemann; 2000:721–731.

Vernick DM. Hearing loss and tinnitus. In: Samuels MA, Feske S, eds. *Office Practice of Neurology*. New York: Churchill Livingstone; 1996:91–98.

Weintraub S. Examining mental state. In: Samuels MA, Feske S, eds. *Office Practice of Neurology*. New York: Churchill Livingstone; 1996: 698–705.

Weiss HD. Dizziness. In: Samuels MA, ed. *Manual of Neurologic Therapeutics*. Boston: Little, Brown & Co.; 1995:58–77.

2

Stroke

Adrian J. Goldszmidt

Anterior Circulation Stroke Syndromes

Affected Vessel	Clinical Features
Middle cerebral artery (MCA)	
Entire territory	Gaze preference (toward lesion), hemiplegia, sensory loss, global aphasia (dominant hemisphere) or neglect (nondominant), hemianopsia; may have depressed level of consciousness
Superior division	Hemiplegia (usually sparing leg), sensory loss, gaze palsy, spatial neglect or Broca's aphasia
Inferior division	Hemianopsia or upper quadrantinopsia, Wernicke's aphasia or constructional dyspraxia
Deep	Hemiplegia, hemisensory loss, transcortical motor and/or sensory aphasia
Anterior cerebral artery (ACA)	
Entire territory	Hemiplegia, abulia, transcortical aphasia (dominant hemisphere), apraxia, ± incontinence
Distal	Weakness of contralateral leg, shoulder weakness, sensory loss, transcortical aphasia
Anterior choroidal	Hemiparesis (face, arm, leg), hemianopia with sparing of horizontal sector; rare neglect, aphasia, or other cortical abnormalities

Distinguishing among different stroke syndromes can be difficult—strokes in different territories often look remarkably similar. Several principles may be helpful: A large vessel cortical stroke is suggested by "cortical signs," such as aphasia, apraxia, agnosia, or neglect. Absence of cortical signs suggests a deep infarct. However, cortical signs may be absent or subtle in large vessel strokes.

Strokes involving vessels that branch from the carotid are termed *anterior circulation* strokes. MCA strokes usually result in weakness involving the face and arm, sparing the leg. ACA strokes involve the leg, not the arm. (Weakness from a posterior cerebral artery stroke is rare.) Deep strokes are more likely to involve the face, arm, and leg equally. A patient with a dense paresis involving the face, arm, and leg with no cortical signs is likely to have a deep stroke.

Pessin, Abbot, and Prager (1986).

Posterior Circulation Stroke Syndromes

Affected Vessel	Clinical Features
Posterior cerebral artery (PCA)	Hemianopsia, hemibody numbness (thalamic perforating vessels fed from proximal PCA), "alexia without agraphia" (left PCA lesion with involvement of splenium of corpus callosum)
Basilar	
Proximal/mid	Quadriparesis (may present asymmetrically), depressed level of consciousness, cranial nerve signs (most commonly extraocular movement abnormalities), "locked-in" syndrome (paralysis of all movement with exception of horizontal eye movements)
Distal ("top of the basilar")	Hemianopsia ± pupillary abnormalities, vertical gaze abnormalities, somnolence, amnesia
Vertebral	Unilateral ataxia; Wallenberg syndrome (infarction of the lateral medulla, usually from stenosis or occlusion of the vertebral artery at the level of PICA, presenting with contralateral pain/temperature loss on body, ipsilateral pain/temperature loss on face, hoarseness and dysphagia, vertigo, and ataxia)

Strokes involving the vertebrobasilar system are termed *posterior circulation* strokes. There are several distinctive features of posterior circulation stroke. Patients with a field cut and awareness of their field cut are likely to have a PCA territory stroke. Absence of awareness of the field cut ("visual neglect" or "spatial neglect") suggests an MCA infarct.

Dense sensory loss involving the trunk suggests a deep (thalamic or spinothalamic tract) infarct, whereas a cortical stroke involving the parietal lobe has sensory loss mainly involving the face and the distal extremities.

Basilar strokes can present asymmetrically, but cranial nerve signs (III, VI, VII) are present almost universally.

Caplan (1989).

Small Vessel Stroke Syndromes

Syndrome	Site (affected vessel)	Symptoms
Pure motor	Internal capsule (lenticulo-striate arteries off proximal MCA) Basis pontis (paramedian pontine perforators)	Motor weakness, usually but not always involving face, arm, and leg equally
Ataxic hemiparesis	Same localization as pure motor, involving fronto-pontine fibers as well as corticospinal fibers	Mild weakness with ipsilateral ataxia
Pure sensory	Thalamus (thalamogeniculate)	Numbness and/or tingling in face, limb, trunk
Sensory/motor	Thalamus/internal capsule (thalamogeniculate)	Hemibody numbness, hemiparesis
Dysarthria/clumsy hand	Dorsal basis pontis (paramedian pontine perforators)	May have associated weakness of face, tongue; findings in arm can be subtle

More than 20 small vessel syndromes have been described. The five listed account for the vast majority of cases seen. Distinguishing between a small vessel stroke and a similar large vessel stroke can be difficult. The following principles make the task easier.

Most small vessel strokes occur in older patients with a history of hypertension. (But note: Emboli and large vessel in-situ thrombus can occlude deep penetrating vessels.) Lenticulostriate infarcts are common in young patients with MCA occlusions and good cortical collaterals. Beware of diagnosing "small vessel disease" in patients without the appropriate risk factors.

Cortical signs (aphasia, neglect, apraxia, agnosia) are rare in small vessel strokes, occurring infrequently when small vessel strokes involve the basal ganglia or thalamus. Involvement of face, arm, *and* leg, especially in the fully conscious patient without cortical signs, makes a cortical stroke (e.g., entire MCA territory) unlikely.

Involvement of the trunk with sensory symptoms makes a thalamic or brainstem localization more likely and a cortical stroke less likely. This is due to the large cortical sensory representation for the face and distal limbs, with relatively little representation of the trunk.

Fisher (1991).

Stroke Risk Factors (by stroke type)

Risk Factor	Thrombosis	Lacune	Embolus	ICH	SAH
Hypertension	++	+++		++	+
Severe HTN		+		++++	++
Coronary disease	+++		++		
Claudication	+++		+		
Atrial fibrillation			++++		
Sick sinus syndrome			++		
Valvular heart disease	+		+++		
Diabetes	+++	+	+		
Bleeding diathesis				++++	+
Cigarette smoking	+++		+		+
Cancer			++	+	+
Old age	+++	+			−
Black or Japanese origin	+	+		++	

HTN: hypertension; ICH: intracerebral hemorrhage; SAH: subarachnoid hemorrhage.

Reprinted with permission from Caplan LR. *Stroke: A Clinical Approach*. 2nd ed. Boston: Butterworth-Heinemann; 1993:76.

Sites of Large Vessel Vascular Disease Causing Stroke

Stroke Mechanism	Site of Vascular Disease
Thrombotic	Anterior circulation (carotid artery) 1. At bifurcation 2. Cervical carotid artery above bifurcation 3. Intracranial carotid artery 4. In-situ MCA, ACA
	Posterior circulation 1. Extracranial subclavian or vertebral arteries 2. Intracranial vertebral artery 3. Basilar artery 4. In-situ PCA
Embolic	Cardiac emboli (see *Cardiogenic Embolic Stroke*) Artery to artery 1. Aortic arch 2. Carotid 3. Proximal vertebral
Other	
Hypoperfusion	Any vessel
Coagulopathy	Any vessel
Arteritis	Any vessel (see *Primary Vasculitides That Affect the Nervous System*, in Chapter 3)

Once a large artery stroke syndrome is diagnosed (on clinical grounds or by imaging), the mechanism usually is found to be either thrombotic or embolic. While there are no hard and fast rules—most patients will have both cardiac and vascular imaging—the following may help guide the workup:

Most embolic strokes are of sudden onset, with maximal deficit at onset.

Most carotid strokes are due to artery-to-artery emboli. Hypoperfusion does not occur until the vessel is 90–95% occluded.

TIAs usually are due to large artery atheroemboli or small vessel disease, rarely from cardiac emboli.

African-Americans and Asians have more intracranial (as opposed to cervical) carotid disease.

Most ACA and PCA strokes are embolic; ACA and PCA stenosis is rare without diffuse atherosclerosis.

Emboli may come from multiple sources.

Martin and Bogousslavsky (1995).

Cardiogenic Embolic Stroke

Nonvalvular atrial fibrillation (NVAF)	Accounts for nearly 50% of cardiogenic emboli. Stroke risk is 6% per year; warfarin cuts this by two-thirds.
Rheumatic heart disease, mitral stenosis	18-fold increased risk of embolic stroke; emboli occur with atrial fibrillation or sinus rhythm
Acute myocardial infarction (MI)	Stroke complicates 2–5% of MI; more common with anterior MI and in first month after MI.
Dilated cardiomyopathy (CM)	Idiopathic CM thought to bear higher risk than ischemic CM. Data supports anticoagulation for reduced ejection fraction (EF) < 20–30%.
Mechanical or prosthetic valves	Incidence of emboli 1–4% per year. Mitral valves more likely to be source of emboli than aortic.
Mitral valve prolapse	Cited as a frequent cause of stroke in the young, but risk is likely quite low (1:6,000 patient-years)
Atrial septal aneurysm (ASA), patent foramen ovale (PFO), atrial septal defect (ASD)	Occurs in up to 35% of the population; ASA often occurs with PFO or ASD. Diagnosis of paradoxical embolism should be made only with presence of right-left shunt *and* existence of venous clot.
Bacterial endocarditis	Stroke occurs in 15–20%, usually within 48 hr of presentation. Anticoagulation not indicated. (See *Neurologic Complications of Infective Endocarditis*, in Chapter 10.)
Nonbacterial thrombotic endocarditis	Can complicate malignancy, AIDS, or connective tissue disorder. Common cause of stroke in patients with cancer.

Distinguishing cardiac embolism from other causes of stroke can be difficult. Classically, emboli present abruptly, but this occurs only 80% of the time. These features suggest cardiogenic embolism: infarcts in multiple territories, emboli to other organs, absence of atherosclerotic disease, hemorrhagic transformation, and "vanishing occlusions" (occlusions seen on an initial angiogram that subsequently disappear).

Strong data support the use of anticoagulation with coumadin for NVAF, rheumatic heart disease, prosthetic valves, dilated cardiomyopathy, and after an acute MI.

The risk of embolization from mitral valve prolapse is low. The risk also is low from atrial septal aneurysms, patent foramen ovale, and ASDs. Strokes secondary to these conditions should not be diagnosed in the absence of thrombus seen on echo, or deep venous thrombosis.

Brickner (1996).

Intracerebral Hemorrhage

Location	Percent of Total	Symptoms
Putamen	33	Contralateral hemiplegia with sensory impairment; hemianopsia, gaze paresis, aphasia, or neglect
Lobar	25	Symptoms similar to those seen in ischemic infarct in same territory
Thalamus	20	Sensory deficits; mild hemiparesis
Cerebellar	8	Ipsilateral ataxia; may have nuchal rigidity or drowsiness progressing rapidly to coma, secondary to brainstem compression
Pontine	8	Quadriplegia, horizontal gaze palsies, pinpoint pupils, coma
Caudate	4	Variable symptoms: can dissect medially into ventricle or laterally, resembling putamenal hemorrhage

Intracerebral hemorrhage (intraparenchymal hemorrhage or subarachnoid hemorrhage) accounts for about 20% of all strokes. The incidence of intraparenchymal hemorrhage is twice that of subarachnoid hemorrhage.

Intraparenchymal hemorrhage can be difficult to distinguish from an ischemic stroke in the same territory. Imaging is required to firmly make the distinction. Headache, nausea, vomiting, and decreased level of consciousness are much more common in hemorrhage than in ischemic stroke.

Goldszmidt and Caplan (1999).

Intraparenchymal Hemorrhage

Cause	Percent of Total	Comments
Hypertension	50–60	Commonly "deep": basal ganglia, thalamus, pons, and cerebellum.
Amyloid angiopathy	10–20	Usually lobar. Incidence increases with age; rare before age 55. MRI may show hemosiderin deposits (evidence of prior bleeds).
Hemorrhagic infarction	10	Risk of hemorrhagic transformation of ischemic infarcts increases with infarct size. Venous infarcts nearly always are hemorrhagic and commonly seen in puerperium.
Anticoagulation or fibrinolysis	10	Risk of hemorrhage on coumadin for atrial fibrillation is 0.3%/year.
Brain tumors	5–10	Especially glioblastoma, metastatic melanoma, ovarian, and renal carcinomas.
Vascular malformation	5	Includes aneurysms, arteriovenous malformations, and cavernous hemangiomas. Consider these especially in younger patients with no other risks. Venous angioma not considered a risk for hemorrhage.
Drugs	<5	Especially sympathomimetics such as cocaine and amphetamines.
Miscellaneous	<5	Includes vasculitis (e.g., polyarteritis nodosa, primary angiitis of the CNS)

Hypertension far and away is the single greatest cause of intracerebral hemorrhage, accounting for 50% of all cases, and the single leading cause for hemorrhage at any location (but especially deep hemorrhages). Two mechanisms are proposed: rupture of small penetrating arteries by chronic hypertension and aging, and sudden blood pressure increases that cause rupture of arterioles unaccustomed to high pressure. Another 25% is attributable to congenital abnormalities, especially aneurysms and AVMs. Lobar hemorrhages in the elderly often are caused by amyloid angiopathy in cortical and leptomeningeal vessels. The incidence of amyloid angiopathy in asymptomatic autopsy series is 37% at age 80. However, hypertension is likely the leading cause of lobar hemorrhage, even in the elderly.

Sacco et al. (1984).

Cause	Comments
Atherosclerotic large vessel disease Hyperlipidemia Juvenile diabetes Homocystinuria Hypertension Radiation therapy	These conditions usually are suggested by a positive family history of early atherosclerosis (hyperlipidemia) or history of the predisposing condition in the patient (e.g., radiation, diabetes, or hypertension). Heterozygotes for homocystinuria rarely have any identifying features, so this disorder should be specifically excluded in young patients with premature atherosclerosis and stroke (see *Inherited Causes of Stroke*).
Nonatherosclerotic disease Dissection Fibromuscular dysplasia Moyamoya disease Vasculitis Takayasu's Polyarteritis nodosa (PAN) Primary angiitis of the CNS	Dissection usually occurs in the setting of trauma but can occur with mild trauma or with no elicitable history. In fibromuscular dysplasia, lesions occur distal to the bifurcations, in locations not typical for atherosclerosis. Takayasu's most commonly occurs in young Japanese women; major pulses will be absent. PAN may have skin lesions (purpuric rash or livedo reticularis) as well as renal involvement. For all these, angiography is crucial to diagnosis. Primary angiitis can cause multiple small infarcts, and angiography can be negative. Brain and leptomeningeal biopsy may be required for diagnosis.
Cardiac embolism Bacterial endocarditis Atrial fibrillation Right-left shunt with DVT Atrial myxoma/tumor	Cardiac sources of emboli are most common in young patients with congenital heart disease, but can occur in other settings. A new murmur, systemic emboli, or fever (with stroke) suggest a cardiac source and possible endocarditis. Transesophageal echocardiography is required to rule out lesions on the mitral valve as well as right-to-left shunting.
Hypercoagulable states Antiphospholipid antibody syndrome (APLAS) Polycythemia vera Essential thrombocytosis Disseminated intravascular coagulation Sickle-cell disease Other coagulopathies (e.g., AT III, protein C or S deficiency)	Clues to a hypercoagulable state may be found in a family history of clotting, previous clotting in the patient, history of spontaneous abortions (for APLAS), or abnormalities on routine bloodwork (RPR, PTT, CBC). Coagulation factor deficiencies (AT III, proteins C and S) are rare causes of arterial thrombosis, usually causing venous thrombosis. Even with "routine" bloodwork and no other diagnostic clues, hypercoagulable states should be ruled out in all young patients with stroke lacking another likely etiology.

AT III: antithrombin III; DVT: deep vein thrombosis; APLAS: antiphospholipid antibody syndrome.

Other causes include cocaine and amphetamines (causing vasospasm, vasculitis, or endocarditis), oral contraceptives, migraine, and genetic causes (see *Inherited Causes of Stroke*).

While the causes of stroke in patients below age 50 often are the same as those for older patients, especially for patients with known risk factors, the history may suggest another diagnosis: trauma in dissection, previous clots in a patient with a clotting disorder. However, no cause is found in as many as 40% of cases.

Stern et al. (1991).

Inherited Causes of Stroke

Disorder	Clinical Features
CADASIL (cerebral autosomal dominant arteriopathy with subcortical infarcts and leukoencephalopathy)	Autosomal dominant disease linked to chromosome 19. Middle-aged adults without usual vascular risk factors present in one of three ways: TIAs and strokes (mainly subcortical), episodic migrainous headache, or psychiatric symptoms, which precede ischemic signs by years. MRI always shows multiple, deep, small infarcts.
MELAS (mitochondrial myopathy, encephalopathy, lactic acidosis, and stroke-like episodes)	90% due to a point mutation in mitochondrial genome. This syndrome is transmitted maternally with onset of symptoms usually by age 15. Patients develop recurrent headaches, strokes with hemianopsia, and cortical blindness. Cortical and subcortical strokes and calcium deposits in basal ganglia are common findings. Ragged red fibers are seen in muscle biopsy.
Homocystinuria	Homocysteine is an intermediate in the metabolism of methionine to cysteine. Excess homocysteine causes focal endothelial loss and fibrosis and premature atherosclerosis. Homozygotes lacking cystathione-beta-synthase have elevated serum methionine and homocysteine levels; they can be developmentally normal or delayed, with bilateral ectopia lentis, retinal detachment, cataracts, and strokes. Heterozygotes for the mutation have elevated homocysteine levels, which have been correlated with increased stroke risk.
Sickle-cell disease	An autosomal recessive hemoglobinopathy. 17% have cerebrovascular symptoms by early adulthood. 75% of symptomatic patients have ischemic strokes, with hemorrhage more frequent in older patients. Most patients have large artery occlusive disease. High blood flow velocity in the MCAs is correlated with increased risk of stroke; transfusion to bring down velocity lowers risk of stroke.
Fabry's disease	A disease of males, caused by X-linked enzyme deficiency in alpha galactosidase A. Ceramide trihexoside accumulates in endothelia and smooth muscle cells, causing multifocal occlusive disease. Multiple infarcts occur in cerebrum, heart, kidneys.

Boers et al. (1985); Baudrimont et al. (1993).

REFERENCES

Baudrimont M, Dubas F, Joutel A, et al. Autosomal dominant leukoencephalopathy and subcortical ischemic stroke. A clinicopathological study. *Stroke*. 1993;24:122–125.

Boers GHJ, Smals AGH, Trijbels FJM, et al. Heterozygosity for homocystinuria in premature peripheral and cerebral occlusive arterial disease. *N Engl J Med*. 1985;313:709–715.

Brickner ME. Cardioembolic stroke. *Am J Med*. 1996;100:465–474.

Caplan LR. Vertebrobasilar system syndromes. In: Vinken PJ, Bruyn GW, Klawans HL, eds. *Handbook of Clinical Neurology*. Vol. 53. Amsterdam: Elsevier Science; 1989:371–408.

Caplan LR. *Stroke: A Clinical Approach*. 2nd ed. Boston: Butterworth-Heinemann; 1993:76.

Fisher CM. Lacunar infarcts—a review. *Cerebrovasc Dis*. 1991;1:311–320.

Goldszmidt AJ, Caplan LR. Intracerebral hemorrhage. In: Rakel R, ed. *Conn's Current Therapy*. Philadelphia: W.B. Saunders Co.; 1999: 882–885.

Martin R, Bogousslavsky J. Embolic versus non-embolic causes of ischemic stroke. *Cerebrovasc Dis*. 1995;5:70–74.

Pessin MS, Abbott BF, Prager R, et al. Clinical and angiographic features of carotid circulation thrombus. *Neurology*. 1986;36.

Sacco RL, Wolf PA, Bharucha NE, et al. Subarachnoid and intracerebral hemorrhage: Natural history, prognosis, and precursive factors in the Framingham Study. *Neurology*. 1984;34:847–854.

Stern B, Kittner S, Sloan M, et al. Stroke in the young. *Maryland Med J*. 1991;40:453–462.

3

Demyelinating and Inflammatory Diseases

George J. Hutton

Signs and Symptoms of Multiple Sclerosis

Motor system	Involvement of corticospinal and corticobulbar pathways leads to upper motor neuron spastic weakness, occurring in up to 80% of patients. This is manifested as spastic paraparesis most commonly, but monoparesis, quadriparesis, or hemiparesis may be seen.
Sensory systems	Sensory complaints occur in up to 75% of patients at some point in the course of the disease and represent the initial manifestation in one-third of patients. The spinothalamic tracts commonly are involved, resulting in dysesthesias. Dorsal column involvement is less common. "Lhermitte's sign" consists of an electric feeling passing down the back to the legs on flexing the neck and occurs in about 40% of patients.
Cerebellar pathways	Ataxia, intention tremor, incoordination, and "scanning" speech indicate cerebellar involvement and tend to occur later in the disease course.
Brainstem	Indicated by nystagmus, diplopia, facial weakness, dysarthria, vertigo, dysphagia, or trigeminal neuralgia. Internuclear ophthalmoplegia (INO) is due to a lesion in the medial longitudinal fasciculus (MLF), causing inability to adduct the ipsilateral eye with nystagmus on abduction of the contralateral eye. Bilateral INO is virtually diagnostic of MS.
Spinal cord	Bowel and bladder dysfunction (urgency and incontinence), sexual dysfunction, and/or autonomic dysfunction commonly are seen.
Optic nerve	Optic neuritis occurs as the initial manifestation in 20% of patients with MS. Patients note unilateral dimming of vision, frequently accompanied by photophobia and pain aggravated by eye movement. Most commonly, patients have a central scotoma and a relative afferent pupillary defect. Fundoscopy reveals a normal appearing optic disc in two-thirds of patients.
Cognitive	Intellectual impairment is common, occurring in up to 60% of patients, in the form of a subcortical dementia. Psychiatric disturbances include depression and psychosis.
Other	Persistent fatigue is a frequent complaint of MS patients, as well as muscle cramps.

Matthews (1998).

Categories of Multiple Sclerosis

Category	Definition	Clinical	Radiology	Treatment
Relapsing remitting (RRMS)	Episodes of acute worsening with recovery and a stable course between relapses. This is the most common pattern at onset but becomes secondary progressive in greater than 50%.	Relapses have an acute or subacute clinical onset during a period of hours or days and usually are self-limited. The disability may resolve partially or almost completely.	T2 hyperintensity from earliest stages of inflammation until the chronic stages. Acute lesions may be surrounded by edema. Acute lesions have disrupted BBB and show enhancement for 2–6 weeks after onset.	Steroids shorten the duration of an attack but do not limit progression. IFN-β-1a (Avonex), -1b (Betaseron), and glatiramer acetate (Copaxone) decrease frequency of attacks. Trials ongoing with IVIG.
Secondary progressive (SPMS)	Gradual neurologic deterioration with or without superimposed acute relapses in a patient who previously had RRMS.	The period of transition from RRMS to SPMS usually occurs after several years, when EDSS is about 4.0.	T2 lesion load increases. Acute lesions as above. Of T2 lesions, 20–30% seen as hypointense on T1 ("black holes"), correlated with axonal loss. MRS shows decreased NAA/creatine and NAA/choline ratios in T2 hyper-intense areas *and* NAWM.	Acute attacks treated with steroids. IFN-β-1b use leads to 20% reduction in disability progression. Other trials ongoing. Symptomatic therapies.
Primary progressive (PPMS)	Gradual, nearly continuous neurologic deterioration from the onset of symptoms. Accounts for 10% of MS cases.	Patients tend to be older at onset (40–60), more likely to be male, and commonly have a progressive myelopathy.	Total area of T2 hyperintensity is less, frequency of new lesions less than in SPMS, but spinal lesions are more common. Enhancement is unusual.	Azathioprine, methotrexate, cyclophosphamide, mitoxantrone, cladribine, cyclosporine, IVIG, plasma exchange, T-cell vaccination.
Progressive relapsing	Gradual neurologic deterioration from the onset of symptoms but with subsequent superimposed relapses. This is a very uncommon pattern.			

IFN: interferon; EDSS: Kurtze's expanded disability status scale; MRS: magnetic resonance spectroscopy; NAA: N-acetyl-aspartate; NAWM: normal appearing white matter; BBB: blood-brain barrier; IVIF: intravenous immunoglobulin.

Tourbah, et al. (1999); Lublin and Reingold (1996); Achiron, et al. (1998); European Study Group on Interferon Beta-1b in Secondary Progressive Multiple Sclerosis (1998).

Diagnostic Criteria for Multiple Sclerosis

Category		Attacks	Clinical Evidence	Paraclinical Evidence	CSF Oligoclonal Bands/IgG
Clinically	CDMS A1	2	2	–	–
definite MS	CDMS A2	2	1 and	1	–
Laboratory-	LSDMS B1	2	1 or	1	+
supported	LSDMS B2	1	2	–	+
definite MS	LSDMS B3	1	1 and	1	+
Clinically	CPMS C1	2	1	–	–
probable MS	CPMS C2	1	2	–	–
	CPMS C3	1	1 and	1	–
Laboratory- supported probable MS	LSPMS D1	2	–	–	+

The clinical definition of MS requires two attacks separated in time and space (i.e., affecting two regions of the body). MS also may be diagnosed on the basis of other combinations of clinical and laboratory evidence. These definitions, shown in the table, are referred to as the *Poser criteria*. Note that *paraclinical evidence* indicates evidence of a subclinical lesion by MRI or evoked potentials. MRI has become the tool of choice in supporting MS diagnoses: Typical white matter lesions are found in up to 97% of those with CDMS. The presence of CSF oligoclonal bands also is a sensitive (found in up to 95% of patients with CDMS) but not specific indicator of MS. See also *Oligoclonal Bands in CSF.*

Reprinted with permission from Poser CM, Paty DW, Scheinberg L, et al. New diagnostic criteria for multiple sclerosis: Guidelines for research protocols. *Ann Neurol.* 1983;3: 227–231.

Fieschi, Gasperini, and Ristori (1997).

Acute Demyelinating Diseases Other Than Multiple Sclerosis

Disease	Clinical Features	Pathology
Neuromyelitis optica (Devic's disease)	Monophasic (35%) or relapsing (55%) disorder characterized by TM and unilateral or bilateral ON. No clinical or radiographic involvement beyond the spinal cord or optic nerves. Two-thirds with poor neurologic outcome, 15% die in the acute stage. CSF with increased protein, pleocytosis but no increase in IgG or oligoclonal bands.	Acute spinal cord lesion shows diffuse swelling and softening, with extensive macrophage infiltration and necrosis of both gray and white matter. Chronic lesions with gliosis, cystic degeneration, cavitation, and atrophy of the spinal cord and optic chiasm. Proliferation of blood vessels with thickened and hyalinized walls is prominent in necrotic areas.
Acute disseminated encephalomyelitis (ADEM)	Monophasic demyelinating disorder following vaccination or infection by 1–6 weeks. More common in children. Course is rapidly progressive, leading to encephalopathy, stupor, coma, seizures, optic neuritis, myelopathy, and brainstem or cerebellar disturbances. Mortality is 10–25%.	Inflammation predominantly in the Virchow-Robinson spaces and diffuse, often symmetric perivenular demyelination. More severe variant is acute hemorrhagic leukoencephalomyelitis (AHLE), in which the inflammatory reaction is associated with perivascular hemorrhages and severe brain edema. ADEM is thought to represent a transient autoimmune response against myelin through molecular mimicry.
Acute transverse myelitis (ATM)	This term usually is reserved for monophasic spinal cord dysfunction. Presents with back pain, ascending sensory level, sphincter disturbance, and paraparesis.	Demyelination or necrosis. May begin as a Brown-Séquard syndrome. Often ascends or spreads transversely. Often spares the posterior columns. Many viral etiologies proposed.
Balo's concentric sclerosis	Monophasic and rapidly progressive, leading to death within a few months. Mostly cerebral symptoms: headache, seizures, aphasia, altered mental status.	Focal necrosis of white matter with mass effect, sparing the cerebellum, brainstem, optic chiasm, and spinal cord. Plaques show alternating rings of myelin preservation and loss, resembling an onion bulb.
Acute MS (Marburg variant)	Severe, nonremitting course with rapid progression to death, usually within one year. Very rare.	Massive macrophage infiltration and acute axonal injury. Small, disseminated lesions in brain and spinal cord may coalesce.

TM: transverse myelitis; ON: optic neuritis.

Lassman (1998); Weinshenker and Lucchinetti (1998).

Diseases That Mimic Multiple Sclerosis

Disease	Similar Features	Unique Features	Laboratory Features
SLE	May present with ON or myelopathy that may be slowly progressive, recurrent, or more commonly, acute or subacute.	Rash, arthralgias. Headache, seizures, encephalopathy more common than in MS.	CSF protein and cells may be higher than expected for MS. CSF OCBs in 42%. TM is strongly associated with aPL antibody. Note: Positive ANA (up to 1:160) in 22% of MS patients.
Behçet's disease	May present with ON or myelopathy. Lhermitte's sign, tonic spasms, and INO do not occur.	Most commonly presents as meningoencephalitis. Oral or genital ulcers, uveitis.	CSF OCB common. CSF may show pleocytosis higher than expected for MS.
Sarcoidosis	May present with ON or myelopathy. Visual loss is usually more gradual than in MS. Lhermitte's sign reported.	More commonly presents as meningoencephalitis. Systemic sarcoid usually present.	CSF with increased protein and cell count. CSF OCB present in 37%. CSF ACE level, CXR, or conjunctival biopsy most diagnostic.
Lyme disease	Cranial nerve signs, spinal cord disease, paresthesias. ON and TM reported.	Rash, constitutional symptoms, endemic areas, tick bite.	CSF may have OCB. Lyme serology in blood and CSF.
Cerebrovascular disease	Multiple emboli from endocarditis, atrial myxoma, etc., may result in clinical picture similar to MS.	Recurrent acute events unusual for MS. Fever, systemic signs of embolic disease.	CSF OCB may be present. Echocardiogram, blood cultures, coagulation studies.
AIDS	Myelopathy combined with dementia may be confused with MS.	Sensory ataxia more common in vacuolar myelopathy of AIDS. Other AIDS-defining illnesses.	CSF OCB rarely present. HIV antibody, viral load, CD4 count.
Meningovascular syphilis	Oculomotor palsies, myelopathy, ON may be confused with MS.	Headache, epilepsy, classical pupillary abnormalities.	Serum RPR, specific treponemal test (MHA-TP), CSF VDRL

TM: transverse myelitis; ON: optic neuritis; CSF: cerebral spinal fluid; INO: internuclear ophthalmoplegia; OCB: oligoclonal bands.

Matthews (1998).

White Matter Lesions on Neuroimaging: Multiple Sclerosis vs. Vascular Etiologies

Disease	Magnetic Resonance Imaging Features
Multiple sclerosis	High SI on T2-WI and PD-WI and intermediate SI on T1-WI. Bilateral, asymmetric distribution of ovoid, periventricular, and corpus callosum lesions. Pontine and midbrain lesions more common than in medulla or cerebellar hemisphere. May cross the midline in the brainstem. Contrast enhancement common.
Vasculitis	Varies from large arterial infarctions to small WM abnormalities or venous thrombosis. WM abnormalities mimicking MS more often seen in SLE, antiphospholipid syndrome, and Behçet's disease.
Systemic lupus erythematosus (SLE)	MRI may mimic MS exactly. However, magnetization transfer ratio (MTR) can help differentiate SLE from MS, as MTR for both lesions and normal appearing white matter (NAWM) are higher in SLE than in MS.
Behçet's disease	Relatively high frequency of selective brainstem and diencephalon involvement.
Migraine	Punctate hyperintense WM lesions on T2-WI and PD-WI in subcortical WM, usually in the frontal lobes. The size, location, and evolution allow differentiation from MS.
Hypertension/ Binswanger's disease	Hyperintensities on T2-WI and PD-WI, with roughly symmetric distribution in subcortical WM. Locations: basal ganglia frequent; corpus callosum rare.
Periventricular leukomalacia (PVL)	Occurs in preterm infants but may not present clinically until adolescence in mildly affected persons. Scattered foci of T2 and PD hyperintensity are visible at the external angles of the lateral ventricles with mild thinning of the periventricular WM.

SI: signal intensity; T2-WI: T2-weighted imaging; PD-WI: proton density weighted imaging; WM: white matter.

Barkhof (1997); Lee et al. (1996); Triulzi and Scotti (1998).

White Matter Lesions on Neuroimaging: Multiple Sclerosis vs. Infectious, Inflammatory, and Metabolic Disorders

Disease	Magnetic Resonance Imaging Features
Lyme disease	MRI may be normal, or show multiple, bilateral hyperintense lesions on T2-WI and PD-WI. Lesions may resemble MS plaques but occur more commonly in the basal ganglia. Lesions tend to be larger than in MS and show peripheral enhancement.
Neurosarcoidosis	May look like MS, but more commonly appears as basal or diffuse granulomatous leptomeningitis with involvement of the optic chiasm, hypothalamus, and pituitary gland seen on T1-WI with contrast.
Progressive multifocal leukoencephalopathy (PML)	Occurs in immunodeficient patients. Lesions occur anywhere in the WM of the cerebral hemisphere, brainstem, and cerebellum. Lesions have intermediate to low SI on T2-WI and PD-WI. Lesions are more confluent than in MS and do not enhance.
HIV encephalitis	Lesions vary from scattered, isolated, unilateral foci to confluent bilateral involvement and may be symmetric or asymmetric. Progressive atrophy and lack of enhancement differentiate this entity from MS.
Subacute sclerosing panencephalitis (SSPE)	Periventricular WM lesions, hyperintense on T2-WI and PD-WI, but more commonly involve the basal ganglia than in MS.
Leukodystrophies	Lesions are usually symmetric, confluent, and progressive. May be confused with MS in initial stages. See *Inherited Leukodystrophy*.
Leukoencephalopathy after radiation or chemotherapy	Periventricular leukoencephalopathy with high signal intensity on T2-WI, PD-WI, and FLAIR sequences. There is no enhancement after contrast is given, and the changes are permanent.

T2-WI: T2- weighted imaging; PD-WI: proton-density weighted imaging; SI: signal intensity; WM: white matter; FLAIR: fluid-attenuated inversion recovery; HIV: human immunodeficiency virus.

Barkhof (1997); Lee et al. (1996); Triulzi and Scotti (1998).

Inherited Leukodystrophy

Disorder	Inheritance	Metabolic Abnormality	Clinical Features
Metachromatic leukodystrophy (MLD)	AR, Chr. 22	Arylsulfatase A (cerebroside sulfatase)	Late infantile form accounts for two-thirds of cases and is most severe. After a period of normal development, gait disturbances develop, followed by hypotonia, then dementia, spasticity, and blindness. Seizures in 50%. Arcuate fibers may be spared on MRI early in the course, frontal demyelinating first. CSF with elevated protein. Peripheral nerves also show demyelination (with slowing on NCS).
Krabbe disease (Globoid cell leukodystrophy)	AR, Chr. 14	β-galacto-cerebrosidase	Early infantile form most common, onset at 3–6 months with restlessness, irritability, and progressive stiffness. Seizures are frequent. MRI with extensive demyelination. Peripheral nerves also show demyelination (with slowing on NCS). CSF with elevated protein. Death occurs by 3–4 years of age.
Adrenoleuko-dystrophy (ALD)	XLR	VLCFA-CoA synthetase	Onset at age 5–8. Behavioral changes, seizures, dementia, optic atrophy, spastic paraplegia. Adrenal insufficiency and bronze skin pigmentation. MRI with demyelination greatest posteriorly, sparing U-fibers. No PNS demyelination. CSF with elevated protein.
Pelizaeus-Merzbacher disease	XLR	Deficient PLP synthesis	Early onset with nystagmus, chorea, athetosis, psychomotor regression after third month. Ataxia and spasticity develop. Optic atrophy and seizures late. Death by age 5–7. NCS and CSF protein normal. MRI with demyelination involving U-fibers.
Canavan disease	AR	Aspartoacylase	Psychomotor arrest and regression during the first 6 months. Decreased awareness, difficulty feeding, irritability, and hypotonia. Later spasticity and megalencephaly are noted. MRI with symmetric demyelination. CSF and NCS are normal.
Alexander disease	Unknown	Unknown	Infantile form most common, with psychomotor retardation, megalencephaly, spasticity, seizures, and death by age 2–3. MRI with demyelination greatest frontally. CSF and NCS normal. Pathology shows Rosenthal fibers.

VLCFA: very long chain fatty acids; PLP: proteolipid protein; PNS: peripheral nervous system.

Fenichel (1997); Aicardi (1993).

Diagnostic Evaluation of Leukoencephalopathy of Unknown Cause

Source	Test	Reason
Blood	ESR, ANA, ANCA, RF, complement	Vasculitis, systemic autoimmune disease
	Coagulation studies	Prothrombotic states: infarction, venous thrombosis
	Vitamin B_{12}, methylmalonic acid	Vitamin B_{12} deficiency
	Lactate, pyruvate, creatine kinase	Mitochondrial encephalopathy
	Serum ACE	Sarcoidosis, Whipple's disease
	Serologies: fungal, HIV, viral, syphilis, cysticercosis	Infection
	Paraneoplastic serologies	Paraneoplastic limbic encephalopathy, encephalomyelitis
	Very long chain fatty acids	Adrenoleukodystrophy
	Arylsulfatase A	Metachromatic leukodystrophy
	DNA mutational analysis	Mitochondrial encephalopathies
CSF	IgG index, oligoclonal bands	MS, SSPE, HIV, other infection
	Measles titer	SSPE
	PCR for *T. whippelii*, JC virus, other viruses	Whipple's disease, PML, viral encephalitis
	Lactate/pyruvate	Mitochondrial encephalopathy
Other	Echocardiogram	Endocarditis, embolic source, PFO
	Angiography	Vasculitis, vasculopathy, atheroembolic disease, venous sinus thrombosis

PFO: patent foramen ovale; PML: progressive multifocal leukoencephalopathy; SSPE: subacute sclerosing panencephalitis.

Weinshenker and Lucchinetti (1998).

Oligoclonal Bands in CSF

Disease	OCB in CSF Only (intrathecal response)	OCB in CSF and Serum, but Different Clones (intrathecal/systemic)	Identical OCB in CSF and Serum (systemic response)
Infectious Viral encephalitis Lyme disease Fungal meningitis Neurosyphilis SSPE or PRP	Yes	Yes	Yes
Inflammatory SLE PSS Behçet's disease Polyarteritis nodosa Sarcoid	Yes	Yes Yes, in 42% Yes, in 37%	Yes
Multiple sclerosis	Yes	Yes, in up to 95% with CDMS	No
Paraneoplastic	Yes	Yes	Yes
Neoplastic	Rare	Rare	Yes
Guillain-Barré syndrome	No	No	Yes
Vascular	No	No	Rare
Degenerative	No	No	Rare

OCB: oligoclonal banding pattern by isoelectric focusing; SSPE: subacute sclerosing panencephalitis; PRP: progressive rubella panencephalitis; PSS: progressive systemic sclerosis; CDMS: clinically definite multiple sclerosis.

In health, CSF contains few immunoglobulins or other plasma proteins. The appearance of immunoglobulin heralds pathological changes, reflecting either increased permeability of the blood-brain barrier or B-cell-related immune processes within the brain parenchyma. An oligoclonal response is defined as the presence of two or more distinct antibody clones, which are apparent because they stand out against the background of *polyclonal* antibody as a result of relatively intense stimulation of a few lymphocyte clones.

OCBs are a nonspecific finding and can be found in the serum or the CSF in response to a number of conditions. The pattern of OCB production and whether the clones are distinct or identical helps narrow the diagnosis. Multiple sclerosis is the most common cause of a mixed "intrathecal/systemic response." Identical OCB in serum and CSF ("systemic response") are seen very rarely in MS and should lead to reconsideration of the diagnosis. Infections and systemic inflammatory disorders can produce any of the three patterns but show the "systemic response" pattern most commonly.

Zeman et al. (1993); Fieschi et al. (1997).

Primary Vasculitides That Affect the Nervous System

Vasculitic Syndrome	Affects CNS	Affects PNS	Autoantibody	Clinical Features
Large vessel				
Giant cell arteritis (temporal arteritis)	++	–		Age >50, new headache, TA tenderness or decreased pulsation, ESR >50 mm/hr, jaw claudication, positive TA biopsy
Primary angiitis of the CNS (PACNS)	++	–		Rare condition with subacute course and varied clinical spectrum, including headache and multifocal signs/symptoms. See *Signs and Symptoms of Primary Angiitis of the CNS*.
Takayasu's disease	++	–	Antiendothelial	Age <40, claudication of limbs, unequal pulses and BP. Affects aorta and its main branches to the limbs and head. Causes syncope, visual changes. TIA/stroke rare. Affects primarily young Asian women.
Medium vessel				
Polyarteritis nodosa	+	++	Hepatitis B	Damage to PNS earlier and more common than to CNS. May cause TIA, stroke, seizures, or encephalopathy. May have intracranial aneurysms. PNS: 60% develop painful MM.
Kawasaki disease	++	–		An acute febrile illness in infants and children of unknown cause. May cause stroke or encephalopathy. Other features are fever, conjunctivitis, lip/oral cavity lesions, rash, and cervical adenitis.
Small vessel				
Churg-Strauss syndrome	+	++	c-ANCA	Asthma, history of allergy, eosinophilia, pulmonary infiltrates, sinusitis. May have stroke, ischemic optic neuropathy, or cerebral hemorrhage. PNS: Up to 60% with painful MM.
Wegener's granulomatosis	+	+	c-ANCA	Oral ulcers, bloody nasal discharge, abnormal CXR, microhematuria. Stroke and basilar meningitis are rare and may be caused by direct invasion from the nasal cavity or vasculitis. PNS: MM or PN.

++: frequent; +: rare; –: not affected; TA: temporal artery; MM: mononeuropathy multiplex; PN: peripheral neuropathy.

Ferro (1998); Younger and Kass (1997).

Secondary Vasculitides That Affect the Nervous System

Vasculitic Syndrome	Affects		Autoantibody	Clinical Features
	CNS	PNS		
Systemic lupus erythematosus (SLE)	++	+	ANA, ds-DNA, anti-SM	CNS involved in up to 75% of SLE with seizures, psychosis, dementia, or stroke. Stroke may be secondary to cardioembolism, prothrombotic state (LA or aCL), vasculopathy, or rarely a true vasculitis. PNS involvement less common with SPN/SMPN or MM.
Rheumatoid arthritis (RA)	+	++	RF	PNS involved more commonly than CNS with SPN/SMPN and MM. CNS involvement may include rheumatoid nodules, meningeal inflammation, and vasculitis.
Sjögren's syndrome	++	++	Anti-SSa/Ro, SSb/La	Primary symptoms are dry eyes and mouth. Focal or diffuse CNS involvement due to antineuronal antibodies or to autoimmune inflammatory cerebral vasculopathy affecting mostly small vessels: focal deficits, seizures, movement disorders, brainstem syndromes, encephalopathy, dementia, or recurrent aseptic meningitis. PNS involvement may include SMPN, SN, or MM.
Behçet's disease	++	+		Presents with uveitis and oral or genital ulcers. Aseptic meningitis or meningoencephalitis occurs in 20%. Focal deficits may occur secondary to ischemia of brain or spinal cord. PNS involvement rare, in the form of SMPN or MM.

++: frequent; +: rare; LA: lupus anticoagulant; aCL: anticardiolipin antibody; SPN/SMPN: sensory/sensorimotor peripheral neuropathy; MM: mononeuropathy multiplex; SN: sensory neuronopathy.

Ferro (1998); Younger and Kass (1997).

Signs and Symptoms of Primary Angiitis of the CNS

Clinical Finding	Percent of Patients
Diffuse cortical dysfunction	95
Headache	68
Focal cerebral dysfunction	50
Evidence of increased intracranial pressure	43
Brainstem or cranial nerve disease	40
Seizures	25
Spinal cord disease	23
Fever or sweats	20
Anorexia or weight loss	20
History and physical examination inadequate for assessment	5

Primary angiitis of the CNS (also known as *granulomatous angiitis*) is a vasculitic syndrome confined to the CNS. It is notoriously difficult to diagnose, because laboratory values (such as ESR) and angiography often are normal, and MRI and CSF usually show nonspecific evidence of inflammation. Brain biopsy may be required for definitive diagnosis. The clinical features listed here derive from a study of 40 patients with histologically confirmed PACNS and represent a subacute encephalopathy, with focal signs of cortical dysfunction appearing gradually, such as hemiparesis, hemianopsia, or seizures. Because of the gradual and nonspecific nature of the syndrome, the mean time from symptom onset to diagnosis has been reported to be six months.

Modified with permission from Vollmer TL, Guarnaccia J, Harrington W, et al. Idiopathic granulomatous angiitis of the central nervous system. *Archiv Neurol.* 1993;50:925–930.

Conditions Mimicking Cerebral Vasculitis

Condition	Examples	Diagnostic Tests
Infection		
Bacterial	Endocarditis, meningitis, syphilis, TB	RPR, HIV, blood and CSF cultures, serologies
Viral	HIV, CMV, Herpes zoster	HIV antibodies, cultures
Fungal	Histoplasmosis, aspergillus	Cultures, serologies
Systemic vasculitis	SLE, Wegener's granulomatosis	H&P, ANA, ANCA
Drugs	Cocaine, amphetamines, ergot	H&P, drug screen
Hematology/ oncology	Intravascular lymphoma	Brain biopsy
	Thrombotic thrombocytopenic purpura	Peripheral blood smear
Vasculopathy	Radiation changes	H&P, angiogram
	Moyamoya/arteriovenous malformations	H&P, angiogram
	Malignant hypertension	H&P
	Vasospasm with intracerebral hemorrhage	MRI, angiogram
	Preeclampsia/puerperium	H&P
	Atherosclerosis	H&P, angiogram
Other	Pheochromocytoma (with hypertension)	H&P, metanephrine screen
	Atrial myxoma	Echocardiogram

H&P: history and physical examination.

Modified with permission from Flynn JA, Hellmann DB. Giant cell arteritis and cerebral vasculitis. In: Johnson RT, Griffin JW, eds. *Current Therapy in Neurologic Disease*. St. Louis: Mosby; 1997:214–219.

REFERENCES

Achiron A, Gabbay U, Gilad R, et al. Intravenous immunoglobulin treatment in multiple sclerosis: Effect on relapses. *Neurology.* 1998;50: 398–402.

Aicardi J. The inherited leukodystrophies: A clinical overview. *J Inherit Metab Dis.* 1993;16:733–743.

Barkhof F. The role of magnetic resonance imaging in diagnosis of multiple sclerosis. In: Thompson AJ, Polman C, Hohlfeld R, eds. *Multiple Sclerosis: Clinical Challenges and Controversies.* St. Louis: Mosby; 1997: 43–63.

European Study Group on Interferon Beta-1b in Secondary Progressive Multiple Sclerosis. Placebo-controlled multicentre randomised trial of interferon beta-1b in treatment of secondary progressive multiple sclerosis. *Lancet.* 1998;352:1491–1497.

Fenichel GM. *Clinical Pediatric Neurology.* Philadelphia: W.B. Saunders Co.; 1997:118–152.

Ferro JM. Vasculitis of the central nervous system. *J Neurol.* 1998;245: 766–776.

Fieschi C, Gasperini C, Ristori G. Differential diagnosis in multiple sclerosis. In: Thompson AJ, Polman C, Hohlfeld R, eds. *Multiple Sclerosis: Clinical Challenges and Controversies.* St. Louis: Mosby; 1997:65–85.

Flynn JA, Hellmann DB. Giant cell arteritis and cerebral vasculitis. In: Johnson RT, Griffin JW, eds. *Current Therapy in Neurologic Disease.* St. Louis: Mosby; 1997:214–219.

Lassman H. Pathology of multiple sclerosis. In: Compston A, Ebers G, Lassmann H, et al., eds. *McAlpine's Multiple Sclerosis.* London: Churchill Livingstone; 1998:323–358.

Lee BCP, Maheshwari M, Zee CS, et al. White matter disease. In: Zee CS, ed. *Neuroradiology.* New York: McGraw-Hill; 1996:309–322.

Lublin FD, Reingold SC. Defining the clinical course of multiple sclerosis: Results of an international survey. *Neurology.* 1996;46:907–911.

Matthews B. Symptoms and signs of multiple sclerosis. In: Compston A, Ebers G, Lassmann H, et al., eds. *McAlpine's Multiple Sclerosis.* London: Churchill Livingstone; 1998:145–190.

Poser CM, Paty DW, Scheinberg L, et al. New diagnostic criteria for multiple sclerosis: Guidelines for research protocols. *Ann Neurol.* 1983;3: 227–231.

Tourbah A, Stievenart JL, Gout O, et al. Localized proton magnetic resonance spectroscopy in relapsing remitting versus secondary progressive multiple sclerosis. *Neurology.* 1999;53:1091–1097.

Triulzi F, Scotti G. Differential diagnosis of multiple sclerosis: Contribution of magnetic resonance techniques. *J Neurol Neurosurg Psych.* 1998;64 (Suppl.):S6–S14.

Vollmer TL, Guarnaccia J, Harrington W, et al. Idiopathic granulomatous angiitis of the central nervous system. *Archiv Neurol.* 1993;50:925–930.

Weinshenker BG, Lucchinetti CF. Acute leukoencephalopathies: Differential diagnosis and investigation. *The Neurologist.* 1998;4:148–166.

Younger DS, Kass RM. Vasculitis and the nervous system. *Neurol Clin.* 1997;15:737–758.

Zeman A, McLean B, Keir G, et al. The significance of serum oligoclonal bands in neurological disease. *J Neurol Neurosurg Psych.* 1993;56: 32–35.

4

Tumors of the Central and Peripheral Nervous Systems

Nicholas P. Poolos

Frequency of Brain Tumors by Age Group

Age Group	Frequency (%)
Children (<15 yr)	
Glioma	61
Craniopharyngioma	11
Germinoma	8
Meningioma	3
Metastatic tumor	3
Other	15
Adult (15–64 yr)	
Glioma	28
Meningioma	21
Pituitary adenoma	15
Metastatic tumor	14
Schwannoma	9
Craniopharyngioma	4
Hemangioblastoma	3
Germinoma	2
Other	5
Elderly (>64 yr)	
Metastatic tumor	31
Meningioma	25
Glioma	23
Pituitary adenoma	7
Schwannoma	7
Other	7

While the frequency of various brain tumors varies among studies, these statistics illustrate some general trends. In children, primary malignant brain tumors by far are the most common; while in adults, metastatic tumors form an appreciable fraction of intracranial neoplasms. Of primary tumors, medulloblastoma and pilocytic (low-grade) astrocytoma are seen predominantly in children, while glioblastoma multiforme and meningioma are rarely seen in those under 20.

Takakura (1995); Lantos, Vandenberg, and Kleihues (1997).

Frequency of Brain Tumors in Adults

Tumor	Percent of Total
Gliomas	45
Glioblastoma multiforme	20
Astrocytoma	10
Ependymoma	6
Oligodendroglioma	5
Medulloblastoma	4
Meningioma	15
Pituitary adenoma	7
Schwannoma	7
Metastatic carcinoma	6
Unclassified (mostly gliomas)	5
Craniopharyngioma, dermoid, epidermoid, teratoma	4
Angioma	4
Sarcoma	4
Miscellaneous (pinealoma, chordoma, granuloma, lymphoma)	3

Statistics about the incidence of intracranial tumors are difficult to obtain, and studies are frequently inconsistent with each other, owing to differing populations sampled, such as tertiary care center vs. community-based sampling. These figures, based on combined series totaling 15,000 patients seen in academic settings, may be taken as a guide to the relative frequencies of the various tumors. The number of metastatic tumors probably is an underestimate of the incidence existing in the community. Also, the incidence of primary CNS lymphoma has increased greatly in recent years owing in part to the increase in numbers of patients with AIDS.

Modified with permission from Adams RD, Victor M, Ropper AH. *Principles of Neurology*. New York: McGraw-Hill; 1997:554.

Frequency of Primary Brain Tumors in Children

Location and Tumor	Percent of Total
Infratentorial	45–60
Primitive neuroectodermal tumor (PNET; medulloblastoma)	20–25
Low-grade astrocytoma, cerebellar	12–18
Ependymoma	4–8
Brainstem glioma	3–9
Low-grade astrocytoma, brainstem	3–6
Other	2–5
Supratentorial hemispheric	25–40
Low-grade astrocytoma	8–20
Malignant glioma	6–12
Ependymoma	2–5
Mixed glioma	1–5
Ganglioglioma	1–5
Oligodendroglioma	1–2
Choroid plexus tumor	1–2
Primitive neuroectodermal tumor (PNET)	1–2
Meningioma	0.5–2
Other	1–3
Supratentorial midline	15–20
Craniopharyngioma	6–9
Low-grade glioma, chiasmatic/hypothalamic	4–8
Germ-cell tumor, suprasellar	1–2
Low-grade glioma, pineal region	1–2
Pituitary adenoma	0.5–2.5
Germ-cell tumor, pineal region	0.5–2
Pineal parenchymal tumor	0.5–2

In contrast to adults, in whom two-thirds of brain tumors are supratentorial, the majority of brain tumors in children are infratentorial, with the most prevalent of these being medulloblastoma and low-grade cerebellar astrocytoma. Low-grade astrocytomas are notable for frequently being completely resectable and thus carrying a favorable long-term prognosis. For children with such a tumor, the 10-year survival is 80–90%.

Modified with permission from Pollack IF. Brain tumors in children. *New Engl J Med.* 1994;331:1500–1507.

Brian Tumors in Adults by Location

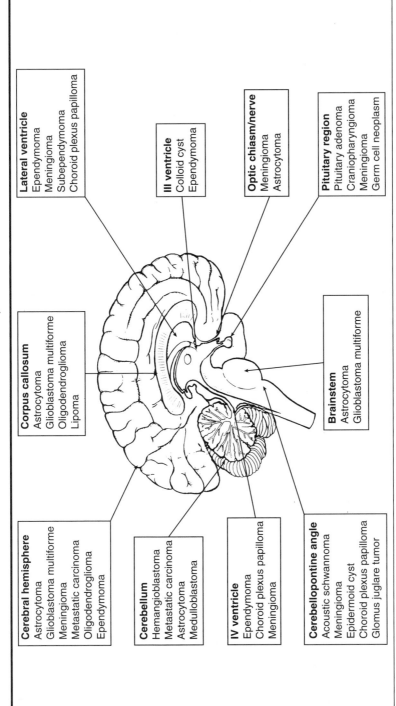

Lateral ventricle
Ependymoma
Meningioma
Subependymoma
Choroid plexus papilloma

III ventricle
Colloid cyst
Ependymoma

Optic chiasm/nerve
Meningioma
Astrocytoma

Pituitary region
Pituitary adenoma
Craniopharyngioma
Meningioma
Germ cell neoplasm

Corpus callosum
Astrocytoma
Glioblastoma multiforme
Oligodendroglioma
Lipoma

Brainstem
Astrocytoma
Glioblastoma multiforme

Cerebral hemisphere
Astrocytoma
Glioblastoma multiforme
Meningioma
Metastatic carcinoma
Oligodendroglioma
Ependymoma

Cerebellum
Hemangioblastoma
Metastatic carcinoma
Astrocytoma
Medulloblastoma

IV ventricle
Ependymoma
Choroid plexus papilloma
Meningioma

Cerebellopontine angle
Acoustic schwannoma
Meningioma
Epidermoid cyst
Choroid plexus papilloma
Glomus juglare tumor

Text outline modified with permission from Burger PC, Scheithauer BW, Vogel FS. *Surgical Pathology of the Nervous System and Its Coverings*. New York: Churchill Livingstone; 1991:144–145. Diagram reprinted with permission from Lippincott.

Brain Tumors in Children by Location

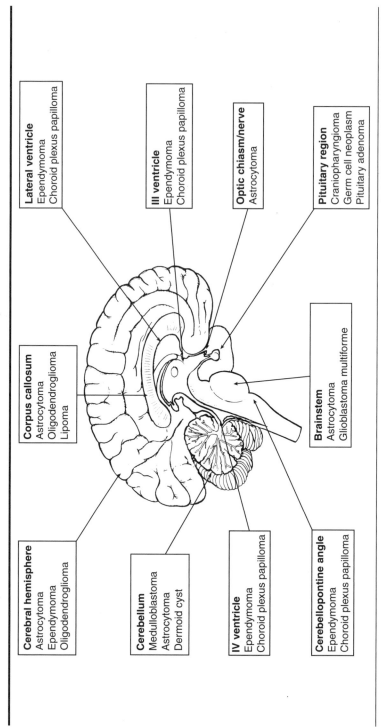

Lateral ventricle
Ependymoma
Choroid plexus papilloma

III ventricle
Ependymoma
Choroid plexus papilloma

Optic chiasm/nerve
Astrocytoma

Pituitary region
Craniopharyngioma
Germ cell neoplasm
Pituitary adenoma

Corpus callosum
Astrocytoma
Oligodendroglioma
Lipoma

Brainstem
Astrocytoma
Glioblastoma multiforme

Cerebral hemisphere
Astrocytoma
Ependymoma
Oligodendroglioma

Cerebellum
Medulloblastoma
Astrocytoma
Dermoid cyst

IV ventricle
Ependymoma
Choroid plexus papilloma

Cerebellopontine angle
Ependymoma
Choroid plexus papilloma

Text outline modified with permission from Burger PC, Scheithauer BW, Vogel FS. *Surgical Pathology of the Nervous System and Its Coverings*. New York: Churchill Livingstone; 1991:144–145. Diagram reprinted with permission from Lippicott.

Common Intraventricular Tumors

	Ventricular Location and Age Group			
Tumor	*Lateral*	*III*	*IV*	*Other Features*
Astrocytoma	All ages	All ages	All ages	May be most common intraventricular tumor
Ependymoma	Adults		Children	Noncommunicating hydrocephalus in children
Choroid plexus papilloma	Children		Adults	Communicating hydro-cephalus due to CSF overproduction
Colloid cyst		Adults		Noncommunicating hydrocephalus, can be intermittent or fulminant
Subependymal giant cell astrocytoma	Child–young adult			Usually calcified and associated with tuberous sclerosis
Meningioma	Adults			Most common extra-axial mass

Woodruff (1993); Schold, Burger, and Mendelsohn (1997).

Clinical Features of Brain Tumors

Tumor	Distinguishing Features
Occurring primarily in adults	
Glioblastoma multiforme, metastatic tumor	Rapid evolution (weeks to months) of headache (worse in A.M. or with recumbency), seizures, nausea or vomiting, papilledema, or focal signs
Astrocytoma (other than glioblastoma), oligodendroglioma	Focal seizures persisting months to years before other signs and symptoms
Meningiomas	
Parasagittal	Slowly progressive (over years) spastic weakness of lower extremities; may present as dementing syndrome
Olfactory groove	Anosmia; ipsilateral optic atrophy, contralateral papilledema (Foster Kennedy syndrome)
Sphenoid ridge	Unilateral exophthalmos
Pituitary adenomas	
Macroadenoma (>1 cm)	Bitemporal hemianopsia; headache; endocrine syndromes (listed below)
Microadenoma (<1 cm)	Endocrine syndromes:
Prolactin	Amenorrhea, galactorrhea
Growth hormone	Acromegaly
ACTH	Truncal obesity, hypertension, hirsuitism, amenorrhea (Cushing disease)
Vestibular schwannoma (acoustic neuroma)	Unilateral hearing loss, tinnitus, accompanying facial weakness or sensory loss
Colloid cyst of III ventricle	Intermittent severe headache with loss of consciousness or lower extremity weakness
Occurring primarily in children	
Ependymoma (of IV ventricle)	Nausea or vomiting, head tilt, gait instability, hydrocephalus; progressive over months to 1–2 yr
Medulloblastoma	Nausea or vomiting, head tilt, gait instability, hydrocephalus; progressive over a few months
Low-grade cerebellar astrocytoma	Slowly progressive gait instability, nausea or vomiting, headache
Craniopharyngioma, other suprasellar lesions	Visual loss plus endocrine disorders: diabetes insipidus, adiposity, slowed physical development

Adams, Victor, and Ropper (1997).

Symptoms and Signs of Brain Tumors

Symptom or Sign	Percent of Total
Headache	57
Nausea	40
Motor weakness	39
Vomiting	31
Cognitive or behavioral change	22
Seizure	19
Visual disturbance	12
Diplopia	8
Cranial nerve VI impairment	7
Cranial nerve V impairment	5
Dizziness or vertigo	5
Ataxia	5

The symptoms of brain tumors vary significantly according to their anatomic location and rate of growth. These statistics were compiled from a study of 204 cases of metastatic tumor and so, while representative of fast-growing intraaxial tumors, may not be representative of other types of primary brain tumors. Note that while headache is the most common presenting sign of an intracranial mass, it is highly nonspecific, with only ~1% of new-onset headache being caused by an underlying mass. The incidence of brain tumor with new onset migraine headache is even less. Therefore, the American Academy of Neurology has adopted the position that routine neuroimaging is not warranted in adult patients with recurrent migraine and no change in headache pattern, history of seizure, or focal neurologic signs or symptoms. No such recommendation was made for patients with headache other than migraine; therefore, when in doubt, neuroimaging always is warranted. See also *Malignant Causes of Headache,* in Chapter 1.

Modified with permission from Takakura K, Sano K, Hojo S, et al. *Metastatic Tumors of the Central Nervous System.* Tokyo: Igaku-Shoin; 1982:128.

Frishberg (1994).

Brain Metastasis

Primary Tumor Type	Percent of Total, Men	Percent of Total, Women
Lung	56	19
Breast	1	53
GI tract	10	6
Prostate	8	—
Urinary tract	7	4
Melanoma	5	5
Head and neck	4	2
Female reproductive organs	—	4
Liver, biliary tract, pancreas	3	2
Thyroid	2	2
Sarcomas	1	3
Others	2	1

Most brain metastasis occurs in patients with evidence of a known primary tumor, most commonly the lung. Metastasis from lung and melanoma have a greater tendency to cause multiple metastases than other primary tumors. (The frequency of lung metastasis cited here may be underestimated due to the recent increased rate of smoking in women.) Hemorrhage in association with an intracranial neoplasm is far more frequent with metastatic than primary brain tumors, but of the latter category, glioblastoma multiforme is the most likely to bleed. Of metastatic tumors, those from primary lung, choriocarcinoma, renal cell, melanoma, and thyroid cancers are the most likely to bleed. Choriocarcinoma may have the greatest tendency to bleed; however, because the lung represents by far the most common source of metastasis to the brain, it accounts for the most cases of metastatic tumors with hemorrhage.

Modified with permission from Takakura K, Sano K, Hojo S, et al. *Metastatic Tumors of the Central Nervous System*. Tokyo: Igaku-Shoin; 1982:13.

Mandybur (1977).

Tumors Affecting the Spinal Cord

Location and Tumor	Clinical Features
Extradural extramedullary	
Epidural metastatic tumor	Back pain (worse in recumbent position, worse with percussion), bilateral lower extremity weakness, bowel and bladder dysfunction
Multiple myeloma	Severe back pain, radicular pain, ± spinal cord involvement; may be associated with cranial or peripheral neuropathy; peak incidence 50–70 years of age
Ewing's sarcoma, neuroblastoma	Common causes of spinal cord compression in children; neuroblastoma most common cause in children <5 yr
Intradural extramedullary	
Schwannoma	Radicular pain due to enlargement of nerve root; pain worsened by Valsalva maneuver; variable spinal cord involvement; most common primary spinal cord tumor; onset 30–60 yr of age.
Meningioma	Radicular pain ± spinal cord involvement; 85% in women, usually in thoracic spine; in men most commonly in cervical spine; multiple meningiomas suggest neurofibromatosis type 2
Leptomeningeal metastasis	Cauda equina syndrome (asymmetrical leg weakness, saddle sensory loss, bowel and bladder dysfunction), cranial neuropathy, and encephalopathy; may have meningeal signs (stiff neck, photophobia); prevalent in association with leukemia and non-Hodgkin's lymphoma
Intramedullary	
Ependymoma	Back pain without sensory loss due to central canal location, or radicular pain and numbness in legs due to cauda equina location; most common intramedullary tumor in adults
Astrocytoma	Back pain and progressive weakness, with variable pace (months to years) depending on tumor grade; most common intramedullary tumor in children
Intramedullary metastasis	Rapidly progressive back pain and weakness, usually localized to thoracic cord; lung, breast, and lymphoma are most common primary carcinomas

Mechtler and Cohen (1996).

Metastatic Causes of Epidural Spinal Cord Compression

Primary Neoplasm Type	Percent of Total
Breast	22
Lung	15
Prostate	10
Lymphoreticular system	10
Sarcoma	9
Kidney	7
Gastrointestinal tract	5
Melanoma	4
Unknown	4
Head and neck	3
Miscellaneous	12

Epidural spinal cord compression occurs in approximately 5% of cancer patients, usually heralded by back pain, followed by weakness, sensory loss, and bowel and bladder incontinence. Epidural metastasis should be strongly considered in any patient with known cancer who presents with new-onset back pain. The need for early diagnosis stems from the observation that, once paraparesis has occurred, it is unlikely to be fully reversed by treatment. The mainstays of acute treatment remain high-dose steroids and X-ray irradiation; surgical intervention usually need not be considered acutely. The data shown here are derived from a study of 583 patients at the Memorial Sloan Kettering Cancer Center. Percentages do not total to 100 due to rounding.

Modified with permission from Posner JB. *Neurologic Complications of Cancer.* Philadelphia: F.A. Davis Co.; 1995:115.

Neurofibromatosis Type 1 vs. Type 2

Feature	Type 1	Type 2
Incidence	1:3,000	1:50,000
Typical tumor	Peripheral nerve neurofibromas, often subcutaneous	Bilateral vestibular schwannomas (acoustic neuromas)
Other tumor types	Optic nerve glioma; ependymoma, astrocytoma, meningioma (less commonly than in type 2)	Ependymoma, astrocytoma, meningioma
Skin lesions	Café au lait spots (six or more >5 mm before puberty is diagnostic); axillary freckling; subcutaneous neurofibromas	Skin lesions are uncommon
Systemic features	Iris hamartomas (Lisch nodules)	None
Cognitive impairment	Frequent, mild	None
Inheritance	Autosomal dominant	Autosomal dominant
Chromosome	Chr. 17	Chr. 22

Neurofibromatosis (NF) is an inherited condition that comprises two diseases with distinct clinical presentations. Type 1 (von Recklinghausen's disease), the more common of the two, is marked by its cutaneous manifestations: pigmented skin lesions (café au lait spots) and peripheral nerve lesions (plexiform neurofibromas), which can become disfiguring as they increase in size and number. Café au lait spots are apparent shortly after birth, but neurofibromas may not become evident until late childhood or adolescence. In contrast, type 2 has few peripheral signs (hence, sometimes referred to as *central* NF) but is defined by the presence of vestibular schwannomas, which eventually occur bilaterally in most patients. Type 2 should be suspected in any patient with bilateral vestibular schwannoma or a family history of unilateral vestibular schwannoma.

Miller and Roach (2000).

Radiologic Features of Brain Tumors

	Margin	Edema	Enhancement	Other Features
Supratentorial hemispheric				
Astrocytomas				
Low-grade	Well defined	–	Little	Discrete mass
Anaplastic	Irregular	+	Irregular	White matter spread
Glioblastoma	Irregular	++	Irregular	Central necrosis; trans-callosal white matter spread
Oligodendroglioma	Well defined	±	Irregular	Calcification in 40%
Metastatic tumor	Well defined	++	Solid, ring	Often multiple, at corti-comedullary junction; edema disproportionate to size of lesion
Meningioma	Well defined	+	Solid	Extra-axial with dural base
Primary lymphoma	Irregular	+	Solid, ring	Diffuse infiltrative or multiple lesions
Supratentorial midline				
Pituitary adenoma	Well defined	–	Solid, cystic	Erosion of sella; displaces optic chiasm
Germinoma	Well defined	–	Solid	Pineal region; ± cystic component
Craniopharyngioma	Well defined	–	Irregular	Suprasellar location; cystic or solid
Infratentorial				
Hemangioblastoma	Well defined	–	Nodular	Cystic cerebellar lesion, mural nodule
Medulloblastoma	Well defined	+	Irregular	Midline cerebellar site in children; lateral in adults
Ependymoma	Well defined	+	Irregular	IV ventricle site
Cerebellar astrocytoma	Well defined	+	Solid or nodular	Solid or cystic with nodule

Schwartz (1995); Woodruff (1993).

REFERENCES

Adams RD, Victor M, Ropper AH. *Principles of Neurology.* New York: McGraw-Hill; 1997:554–598.

Burger PC, Scheithauer BW, Vogel FS. *Surgical Pathology of the Nervous System and Its Coverings.* New York: Churchill Livingstone; 1991: 144–145.

Frishberg BM. The utility of neuroimaging in the evaluation of headache in patients with normal neurologic examinations. *Neurology.* 1994; 44:1191-1197.

Lantos PL, Vandenberg SR, Kleihues P. Tumours of the nervous system. In: Graham DI, Lantos PC, eds. *Greenfield's Neuropathology.* New York: Oxford University Press; 1997:584.

Mandybur TI. Intracranial hemorrhage caused by metastatic tumors. *Neurology.* 1977;27:650–655.

Mechtler L, Cohen ME. Clinical presentation and therapy of spinal tumors. In: Bradley WG, Daroff RB, Fenichel GM, Marsden CD, eds. *Neurology in Clinical Practice.* 2nd ed. Boston: Butterworth-Heinemann; 1996: 1150–1159.

Miller VS, Roach ES. Neurocutaneous syndromes. In: Bradley WG, Daroff RB, Fenichel GM, Marsden CD, eds. *Neurology in Clinical Practice.* 3rd ed. Boston: Butterworth-Heinemann; 2000:1665–1700.

Pollack IF. Brain tumors in children. *New Engl J Med.* 1994;331:1500–1507.

Posner JB. *Neurologic Complications of Cancer.* Philadelphia: F.A. Davis Co.; 1995:115.

Schold SCJ, Burger PC, Mendelsohn DB. *Primary Tumors of the Brain and Spinal Cord.* Boston: Butterworth-Heinemann; 1997:84.

Schwartz RB. Neuroradiology of brain tumors. *Neurol Clin.* 1995;13: 723–756.

Takakura K. Metastatic brain tumours. In: Thomas DGT, Graham DI, eds. *Malignant Brain Tumours.* London: Springer-Verlag; 1995:171–192.

Takakura K, Sano K, Hojo S, et al. *Metastatic Tumors of the Central Nervous System.* Tokyo: Igaku-Shoin; 1982;13:128.

Woodruff WW. *Fundamentals of Neuroimaging.* Philadelphia: W.B. Saunders Co.; 1993:71–120.

5

Epilepsy

Nicholas P. Poolos

Classification of Seizures

Seizure Type	Clinical Features
Simple partial	Begins on one side of the body and does not impair consciousness. May have motor (clonic or tonic movements) or sensory (paresthesias, visual hallucinations) manifestations. Ictal EEG usually shows a contralateral focal discharge.
Complex partial	As typically seen in temporal lobe epilepsy, there is impairment of consciousness, along with automatisms (chewing, picking at clothes). Often preceded by an aura of olfactory or visceral sensations, or a sensation of false memory (déjà vu). A postictal phase is common and may last minutes to hours. Ictal EEG usually demonstrates unilateral or bilateral temporal discharges. (Complex partial seizures also may emanate from the frontal lobes.)
Absence	Sudden onset of unresponsiveness lasting seconds, with interruption of ongoing activity but no loss of muscle tone. On cessation of the seizure, patient returns to previous activities with no postictal phase. Ictal EEG shows generalized 3 Hz spike and waves.
Tonic-clonic	Sudden loss of consciousness with onset of rigid muscle tone (tonic phase) followed by rhythmic convulsive movements lasting up to several minutes (clonic phase). Some patients experience a brief prodromal vague sensation. Postictal somnolence lasts for minutes to a few hours. Ictal EEG shows bilateral 10 Hz activity (tonic) followed by slow waves or sharp and slow wave complexes (clonic).
Myoclonic	Brief contractions of trunk or extremities without loss of consciousness, often occurring at sleep onset and on awakening. These attacks must be distinguished from other forms of myoclonus. Ictal EEG shows generalized polyspike and waves.
Atonic	Sudden loss of axial muscle tone, causing precipitous falls, and often, head injury. Ictal EEG shows generalized polyspike and waves or low-voltage fast activity.

Seizures are classified by their site of onset: *partial,* if localized to one cerebral hemisphere; *generalized,* if simultaneously in both hemispheres. Seizures of partial onset may spread to the other side, or *secondarily generalize.* Partial seizures that do not affect consciousness are *simple,* whereas those that do are *complex.* Warning signs or symptoms are termed an *aura,* and alterations of consciousness following a seizure constitute a *postictal* state.

Dreifuss (1997).

Absence vs. Complex Partial Seizures

Feature	Absence	Complex Partial
Age of onset	Usually childhood	Usually teens to early adult
Seizure duration	Seconds	Seconds to several minutes
Aura	None	Frequent olfactory or visceral or emotional sensations
Postictal phase	None	Usual; may be prolonged
Automatisms	Often	Often
Provoked by hyperventilation	Common	Uncommon
EEG (interictal)	Generalized 3 Hz spike and wave	May be normal or with focal (usually temporal) spikes, sharp waves, or slowing
MRI	Normal	May be abnormal (focal lesion or mesial temporal sclerosis)
AED response	Good to ETX, VPA	May be resistant

VPA: valproate; ETX: ethosuximide.

Complex partial seizures, which can appear as brief periods of unresponsiveness, frequently are confused with absence seizures and often mislabeled with the older term, *petit mal*. These two entities, which have markedly different treatments and prognoses, often can be distinguished by history; in particular, the presence of an aura or a postictal state is the feature from the history that most reliably differentiates the two causes. As a rule, adults with brief periods of unresponsiveness due to epilepsy are much more likely to have complex partial seizures than absence seizures as the underlying etiology.

Guberman and Bruni (1999).

Localization of Partial Seizure Focus by Clinical Features

Location	Clinical Features
Temporal lobe	Gradual evolution. Auras, especially olfactory, gustatory, or gastrointestinal sensations. Affective symptoms may be present as may be dysmnesic symptoms, such as déjà vu. Automatisms are nonviolent (lip smacking, fidgeting). Prominent postictal confusion. About 60% of complex partial epilepsy syndromes.
Frontal/precentral	Clonic and dystonic movements in contralateral extremity with "Jacksonian march" (spread to contiguous body parts over seconds). Head initially turns away from side of ictal onset. Postictal (Todd's) paralysis in an extremity may occur.
Frontal/supplementary motor	Brief episodes of abnormal posturing of extremities, usually with consciousness preserved. Abrupt onset, often in clusters, occurring in sleep. Automatisms can be violent and mistaken for psychogenic seizures, such as bilateral bicycling and kicking movements without loss of consciousness. Little postictal confusion.
Parietal lobe	Somatosensory symptoms and illusions.
Occipital lobe	Elementary visual hallucinations, usually of multicolored circular shapes and patterns. Their qualities differ from the visual phenomena of migraine, which are more likely to be angular shapes (e.g., "fortifications") and white or uncolored.
Dominant hemisphere for language	Ictal speech arrest in ~two-thirds of patients with temporal lobe epilepsy.
Nondominant hemisphere for language	Ictal preservation of speech in ~80% of patients with temporal lobe epilepsy.

The localization of a seizure focus is an imprecise art when based on seizure semiology. One difficulty, especially with temporal lobe epilepsy, is to predict which temporal lobe is acting as the initial locus of seizure onset. While EEG monitoring always is necessary to make a firm identification of the site and side of seizure onset, several clinical features may be predictive of the side of temporal lobe onset: unilateral motor manifestations (jerking, dystonic posturing) and tonic head deviation to one side usually indicate a contralateral focus; preservation of speech during a seizure strongly predicts onset in the nondominant hemisphere (speech arrest, however, is not as predictive of dominant hemisphere onset).

Walker and Shorvon (1997); Marks and Laxer (1998).

Common Epileptic Syndromes

Syndrome	Seizure Appearance	Aural/Postictal State	Onset/Remission	AED Response	EEG (interictal)
Infantile spasms	Myoclonic, with extensor or mixed flexor/extensor spasms of trunk and extremities	None/Infant may be irritable after seizure	2 wk–2 yr, most have onset before first year of life/ Remission depends on etiology	Variable response to VGB, ACTH, or prednisone; long-term outcome depends on underlying etiology	Hypsarrhythmia is usual pattern; may have a variety of other patterns, including normal background
Febrile seizures	GTC lasting <15 min with fever; *complex* febrile seizures have focal features and longer duration	Unclear/May have brief lethargy but not focal deficits in *simple* febrile seizures	6 mo–3 yr; peak incidence 18–24 mo/Usually remits by 5 yr	AEDs may be unnecessary, as only ~10% have more than two seizures; antipyretics may help	Nonspecific generalized abnormalities, or may be normal
Childhood absence epilepsy	Brief staring spells, often with automatisms	None/None	3–7 yr, usually in teens	Good to ETX, VPA	Generalized 3 Hz spike and wave
Juvenile myoclonic epilepsy	Myoclonic jerks on awakening, most with GTC or absence seizures as well	None/None after myoclonic seizures	10–25 yr/Does not remit	Usually responds well to ETX, VPA	Generalized 3.5–4 Hz spike and wave
Benign Rolandic epilepsy (BCETS)	Facial twitching, speech arrest, with nocturnal GTC	Variable unilateral facial paresthesias/Rare postictal phase	Usually 5–10yr/ Remits in teens	Excellent	Spike and slow waves in central (Rolandic) areas; may be bilateral
Temporal lobe epilepsy	Staring spells, automatisms, often followed by GTC	Visceral sensations, déjà vu, lasting secs to 1–2 min/Often prolonged postictal phase	Teens–20s/Usually does not remit	Often resistant	None or temporal spikes, slowing

AED: antiepileptic drug; GTC: generalized tonic-clonic [seizures]; BCETS: benign childhood epilepsy with centrotemporal spikes; VGB: vigabatrin; ETX: ethosuximide; VPA: valproate.

Holmes (1997); Guberman and Bruni (1999); Duchowny (1996).

Etiology of Epilepsy by Age Group

	Children (<15 yr)	Young Adults (15–34 yr)	Adults (35–64 yr)	Elderly (>64 yr)
Idiopathic	68	84	55	49
Congenital	20	3	—	—
Traumatic	5	5	10	3
Infectious	4	3	2	1
Neoplastic	2	3	11	3
Degenerative	1	1	3	12
Vascular	—	—	16	32

Etiology as a percentage of the total for each age group.

The data shown here derive from the Rochester (Minnesota) Epidemiology Project, which has tracked the medical diagnoses of residents of Olmsted County, Minnesota, since 1935. Although in all age groups the underlying cause of epilepsy most commonly is never determined, there is a pattern to the next most common diagnoses. In children, congenital causes are common, such as tuberous sclerosis, migrational disorders, or other structural abnormalities of the brain. In the elderly, stroke is a frequent cause of new-onset seizures. The middle-aged adult who develops epilepsy, however, always should raise suspicion of an underlying brain tumor. Percentages may not total to 100 due to rounding.

Modified with permission from Hauser WA. Seizure disorders: The changes with age. *Epilepsia.* 1992;33:S6–S14.

Annegers, Rocca, and Hauser (1996).

Inherited Epilepsy Syndromes

Benign familial neonatal convulsions

A rare syndrome consisting of generalized seizures usually beginning in the first few days of life and usually remitting within six weeks. The interictal EEG and cognitive development are normal in most children. Inheritance is autosomal dominant with high penetrance and is related to mutations in either of two potassium channel genes (KCNQ2 and KCNQ3) on chromosomes 20 and 8.

Childhood absence

Generalized absence seizures with onset from 4–8 years of age associated with a 3 Hz spike-and-wave EEG. Inheritance most likely is polygenic, with the risk of epilepsy in a first-degree relative around 30% (higher if an abnormal EEG is used as the criteria for affectedness).

Juvenile myoclonic epilepsy

Myoclonic seizures, usually of upper extremities, occurring in the early morning, with onset in the teens; most patients also have generalized tonic-clonic (GTC) and absence seizures. The EEG shows generalized 3.5–4 Hz spike and waves. Although this is a common epilepsy syndrome (up to 10% of all epileptic patients), it is significantly underdiagnosed, especially if GTC seizures are infrequent. The mode of inheritance is unclear, with some studies suggesting a link to chromosome 6. Up to 12% of first-degree relatives may demonstrate an abnormal EEG.

Benign childhood epilepsy with centrotemporal spikes (BCETS)

Also known as *benign Rolandic epilepsy*. Seizures typically consist of unilateral facial twitching and speech arrest with preserved consciousness. The EEG shows interictal spikes in the centrotemporal region. Onset is after 4 years, with resolution by the teens. Inheritance appears to be autosomal dominant with incomplete penetrance; one study found seizures in 11% of siblings, with centrotemporal EEG abnormalities in 34%.

Myoclonus epilepsy with ragged red fibers (MERRF)

A syndrome characterized by myoclonus epilepsy, ataxia, myopathy, and progressive dementia. The clinical presentation is quite varied, even within the same family, but symptoms usually have their onset in the second decade. Inheritance is maternal, via mitochondrial DNA, and has been found to be a base pair substitution in most kindreds.

Biervert et al. (1998); Buchhalter (1994); Elmslie and Gardiner (1997).

Status Epilepticus

Etiology	Percent of Total	Percent "Good" Outcome
Anticonvulsant withdrawal	25	89
Alcohol related	25	89
Drug toxicity	9	70
CNS infection	8	66
Refractory epilepsy	6	78
Trauma	5	100
Unknown	5	64
CNS tumor	5	57
Metabolic disorder	3	32
Stroke	3	32
Cardiac arrest	3	20

This information was compiled in a retrospective study of admissions for status epilepticus to San Francisco General Hospital from 1980–1989. The primary probable cause of status epilepticus is listed; some patients had other contributing causes. A *good* outcome was defined as discharge from the hospital with either a mild or no neurological deficit. In this study, 44% of the patients had no prior history of seizures, and in this group the most common causes of new-onset status epilepticus were alcohol related, 21%; drug toxicity, 18%; and CNS infection, 15%.

Lowenstein and Alldredge (1993).

Lesional Causes of Intractable Epilepsy

Pathology	Frequency (%)
Low-grade tumors	31
Astrocytoma, ganglioglioma, oligodendroglioma, hamartoma	17
Dysembryoplastic neuroepithelial tumor (DNET)	7
Meningioma	6
Epidermoid cyst	1
Neuronal migration disorders	29
Subcortical heterotopia	21
Pachygyria, polymicrogyria	8
Vascular malformations	20
Cavernous angioma	13
Arteriovenous malformation (AVM)	8
Gliotic lesions due to an early insult (e.g., prenatal infarction)	10
Porencephalic cysts	10

A subset of patients with intractable epilepsy of partial onset will have an identifiable lesional cause. The identification of potentially surgically treatable lesions has increased markedly with the widespread adoption of improved neuroimaging techniques and therefore mandates use of MRI in virtually all patients with epilepsy (with usual exception of children with absence epilepsy).

Mesial temporal sclerosis per se is not included here as a lesional etiology, although Cendes et al. (1995) show that 15% of patients with an identifiable lesion also will have mesial temporal sclerosis ("dual pathology"). Some studies of chronic epilepsy in developing countries have found that cysticercosis is a significant etiology, perhaps accounting for 20–30% of epilepsy in countries where cysticercosis is endemic. Percentages may not add correctly due to rounding.

Cendes et al. (1995); Garcia et al. (1993).

Progressive Myoclonus Epilepsy

Disease	Age at Onset (yr)	Clinical Features	Laboratory Features
Unverricht-Lundborg disease	8–13	Severe myoclonus with little or no dementia	Mutation in cystatin B gene (Chr. 21)
Lafora-body disease	11–18	Occipital seizures with progressive dementia	Lafora bodies on skin or other organ biopsy
Neuronal ceroid lipofuscinosis (NCL)			
Late infantile	2.5–4	Severe epilepsy, rapid regression, macular degeneration	All NCLs marked by inclusions in skin or brain biopsy
Juvenile	4–10	Visual loss and macular degeneration	
Adult	12–50	Psychiatric disorders, cognitive decline	
Sialidosis			
Type I	8–20	Severe myoclonus, cherry-red spot in fundus	Both type I and II marked by elevated urinary oligosaccarhrides and neuraminidase deficit in fibroblasts
Type II	10–30	Cherry-red spot	
MERRF	5–40s	Short stature, hearing loss	Ragged red fibers on muscle biopsy; abnormal mitochondrial DNA analysis

MERRF: Myoclonus epilepsy and ragged red fibers.

The progressive myoclonic epilepsies are uncommon disorders characterized by myoclonic and tonic-clonic seizures and progressive neurological deterioration. The myoclonic seizures generally begin in childhood or young adulthood, and the presence of accompanying neurological (usually cognitive) decline distinguishes these syndromes from the more common juvenile myoclonic epilepsy. Only the most frequent causes are listed here. All, with the exception of MERFF, are transmitted by autosomal recessive inheritance (MERFF is predominantly maternally inherited). Definitive diagnosis is often dependent on demonstrating characteristic intracellular inclusions or enzymatic defects.

Modified with permission from Berkovic SF, Andermann F, Carpenter S, Wolfe LS. Progressive myoclonus epilepsies: Specific causes and diagnosis. *New Engl J Med.* 1986;315:296–303.

Delgado-Escueta, Serratosa, Medina (1996).

Paroxysmal Events That Resemble Epilepsy in Children and Adults

Event	Distinguishing Features
Cardiogenic syncope	Sudden loss of consciousness without stereotypical convulsions. Palpitations may occur, or EKG may be abnormal. Should be suspected in any patient, especially middle-aged or elderly, with cardiac risk factors. See also *Syncope vs. Seizure*, in Chapter 1.
Noncardiac syncope	Aura of lightheadedness and slow loss of postural tone in orthostatic syncope. Vasovagal syncope may be precipitated by emotional stimulus, cough, or urination (micturition syncope in men).
Breath-holding spells	Loss of consciousness and color change in children provoked by an episode that makes the child cry. The color change precedes the loss of consciousness. Usually starts at 6–28 months of age and is rare after 5 or 6 years of age.
Benign paroxysmal vertigo	Retained consciousness in child who is frightened and exhibits disequilibrium.
Paroxysmal dyskinesia	Paroxysmal bouts of choreiform or athetoid movements, without loss of consciousness, typically in children or teenagers. May be precipitated by movement or startle and occur many times a day. See also *Paroxysmal Movement Disorders*, in Chapter 6.
Confusional migraine	Prolonged prodrome (>5 min) of altered consciousness but rarely does frank loss of consciousness occur. A postdromal headache follows. Usually occurs in children and adolescents.
Psychogenic seizure (pseudoseizure)	Some features include lack of EEG changes during episode, violent thrashing movements rather than tonic-clonic movements, prolonged course, retained consciousness despite bilateral motor manifestations. See also *Features of Psychogenic Seizures (Pseudoseizures)*.

Morrell (1993); Murphy and Dehkharghani (1994).

Features of Psychogenic Seizures (Pseudoseizures)

Clinical Feature	Caveat
Gradual onset of seizure	Epileptic seizures begin suddenly but often are preceded by auras (<2 min) or premonitory symptoms (minutes or hours)
Prolonged duration	Epileptic seizures usually last <4 min, but must distinguish between ictal and postictal state
Thrashing, struggling, crying, pelvic thrusting, side-to-side rolling	Bizarre automatisms may be seen with frontal lobe complex partial seizures
Motor activity starts and stops	Activity that waxes and wanes several times during the same spell is very rare in epilepsy
Intermittent, arrhythmic, out-of-phase jerking	During GTC seizures, jerking is rhythmic and in-phase; frontal lobe seizures may be an exception
Bilateral motor activity with preserved consciousness	May occur with supplementary motor area (frontal lobe) seizures
Ability to talk during bilateral tonic or clonic movements	Automatic speech may occur during complex partial seizures
Clinical features that fluctuate from one seizure to the next	Epileptic seizures usually are stereotypic
Postictal crying or shouting obscenities	Aggressive verbal and physical behavior can occur if patients are restrained
Lack of postictal confusion or lethargy after CP or GTC seizures	May occur with frontal lobe and, less often, temporal lobe CP seizures
Suggestibility (ability to talk someone into or out of a seizure or produce a seizure with provocative tests such as saline induction)	(No caveat)

While the only reliable means of distinguishing between epileptic and nonepileptic (psychogenic or pseudoseizure) seizures depends on video-EEG monitoring of a typical attack, a number of clinical features are typical of psychogenic seizures. Note, however, that many of these features can be seen less commonly in epileptic seizures.

Modified with permission from Devinsky O, Thacker K. Nonepileptic seizures. *Neurol Clin.* 1995;13:299–319.

Seizures in Neonates

Cause	Percent of Total
Hypoxic-ischemic encephalopathy (HIE)	32
Intracranial hemorrhage	17
CNS infection	14
Cerebral infarction	7
Chromosomal abnormality/cerebral dysgenesis	7
Hypocalcemia	4
Inborn errors of metabolism	3
Neurodegenerative disorders	3
Hypoglycemia	2
Benign neonatal convulsions	2
Unknown	9

The most common cause of seizures in neonates is HIE, which results from intrauterine asphyxia, with seizures usually presenting within the first 12 hours of life. Intracranial hemorrhage often results from birth trauma in primiparous mothers, with the exception of intraventricular bleeds in premature infants. CNS infections tend to present with seizures in the first 24 hours, with the exception of herpes simplex, which usually presents after the first week. Inborn errors of metabolism present with seizures and lethargy after the first 48 hours of life, once the infant has begun to feed. Pyridoxine dependency, while a rare occurrence and not listed separately here, always should be considered in cases of intractable neonatal seizures.

Modified with permission from Mizrahi E, Kellaway P. *Diagnosis and Management of Neonatal Seizures.* Philadelphia: Lippincott-Raven; 1998:52.

Fenichel (1997).

Myoclonic Seizures in Infants

Clinical Features	Characteristic Interictal EEG
Infantile spasms	
Clusters of flexor or mixed flexor-extensor movements involving the trunk, limbs, and neck, generally appearing around 4–7 months of age. Specific etiology may be found in 75%, including tuberous sclerosis or congenital malformations. Pyridoxine or biotinidase deficiency is a rare cause.	Hypsarrhythmia; but also slow spike and wave, burst suppression, focal or multifocal spikes, diffuse or focal slowing; rarely normal
Severe myoclonic epilepsy	
A progressive seizure disorder initially presenting as generalized or focal seizures, often febrile, then progressing to myoclonic seizures after 1 year of age. Seizures are accompanied by progressive neurologic deterioration. Positive family history of epilepsy in 25% of cases.	Polyspike and wave, >3 Hz
Benign myoclonic epilepsy	
Rare presentation of myoclonic seizures in which brief bouts of myoclonus are accompanied by preservation of consciousness. Onset is 4 months to 2 years of age, with no signs of neurologic decline. About one-third of patients have a positive family history for epilepsy.	Polyspike and wave, 3 Hz
Benign myoclonus of infancy	
Appearing similar to infantile spasms, yet with a normal ictal EEG. Symptoms usually spontaneously resolve after several months with no neurologic sequelae.	Normal

Fenichel (1997).

Childhood Epilepsy with Developmental Regression

West syndrome

Infantile spasms (rapid flexion or extension of the trunk and/or extremities followed by a tonic phase lasting a few seconds) in association with developmental regression and hypsarrhythmia on EEG. This syndrome usually begins around 4 months of age and rarely after 18 months. Multiple underlying causes include tuberous sclerosis and cortical migrational disorders, and the long-term outcome depends strongly on the etiology. Treatment consists of ACTH, prednisone, or vigabatrin.

Lennox-Gastaut syndrome

Consists of a triad of seizures (atypical absence, atonic, and axial tonic seizures), with other seizure types as well. The EEG has the hallmark feature of slow spike and wave (1.5–2.5 Hz). This syndrome has its onset in childhood, usually in previously developmentally delayed children, and has a dismal prognosis. The seizures are difficult to control, usually requiring multiple agents; the atonic seizures, in particular, pose a significant risk of head trauma to the patient.

Landau-Kleffner syndrome

Also known as *acquired epileptic aphasia*, this syndrome consists of seizures that begin in a previously normal child, associated with loss of receptive language. The developmental regression ultimately may come to resemble autism, sometimes resulting in misdiagnosis. Unlike autism, however, premorbid language development in the child is normal and, in some cases, has been restored by administration of steroids. The seizure disorder usually is well-controlled with anticonvulsants.

Epilepsy with continuous spike and wave during slow-wave sleep (electrical status epilepticus during sleep; ESES)

Seizures—virtually continuous electrographic activity—occur during slow-wave sleep. Developmental regression also occurs, particularly in language, leading some to suggest that ESES and Landau-Kleffner represent points on a continuum of degenerative epilepsies. Seizures during sleep usually are resistant to treatment.

Rasmussen's syndrome

An inflammatory encephalopathy affecting usually one cerebral hemisphere, associated with intractable seizures and hemiparesis on the affected side. The onset usually is between 14 months and 14 years and clinically resembles a viral encephalitis. Laboratory evidence suggests that an autoimmune response against glutamate receptors may underlie the disease. Hemispherectomy is the only treatment of proven benefit, although immunotherapy may help.

Progressive myoclonus epilepsies

A heterogeneous group of progressive dementing disorders associated with myoclonic epilepsy. Age of onset can range from late infancy to middle age. The underlying disorders include storage diseases, mitochondrial disease, and other genetic causes. See *Progressive Myoclonus Epilepsy*.

Dreifuss (1997).

REFERENCES

Annegers J, Rocca WA, Hauser WA. Causes of epilepsy: Contributions of the Rochester Epidemiology Project. *Mayo Clin Proc.* 1996;71:570–575.

Berkovic SF, Andermann F, Carpenter S, Wolfe LS. Progressive myoclonus epilepsies: Specific causes and diagnosis. *New Engl J Med.* 1986;315: 296–303.

Biervert C, Schroeder BC, Kubisch C, et al. A potassium channel mutation in neonatal human epilepsy. *Science.* 1998;279:403–406.

Buchhalter J. Inherited epilepsies of childhood. *J Child Neurol.* 1994;9: S12–S19.

Cendes F, Cook MJ, Watson C, et al. Frequency and characteristics of dual pathology in patients with lesional epilepsy. *Neurology.* 1995;45:2058–2064.

Delgado-Escueta AV, Serratosa JM, Medina MT. Myoclonic seizures and progressive myoclonus epilepsy syndromes. In: Wyllie E, ed. *The Treatment of Epilepsy: Principles and Practice.* Baltimore: Williams & Wilkins; 1996:467–483.

Devinsky O, Thacker K. Nonepileptic seizures. *Neurol Clin.* 1995;13: 299–319.

Dreifuss FE. Malignant syndromes of childhood epilepsy. In: Porter RJ, Chadwick D, eds. *The Epilepsies*, Vol. 2. Boston: Butterworth-Heinemann; 1997:157–166.

Dreifuss FE. Classification of epileptic seizures. In: Engel J, Pedley TA, eds. *Epilepsy: A Comprehensive Textbook.* Philadelphia: Lippincott-Raven; 1997:517–524.

Duchowny M. Febrile seizures in childhood. In: Wyllie E, ed. *The Treatment of Epilepsy: Principles and Practice.* Baltimore: Williams & Wilkins; 1996.

Elmslie F, Gardiner RM. Epilepsy and the new genetics. In: Porter RJ, Chadwick D, eds. *The Epilepsies.* Boston: Butterworth-Heinemann; 1997:49–70.

Fenichel GM. *Clinical Pediatric Neurology.* Philadelphia: W.B. Saunders Co.; 1997:1–46.

Garcia HH, Gilman R, Martinez M, et al. Cysticercosis as a major cause of epilepsy in Peru. *Lancet.* 1993;341:197–200.

Guberman AH, Bruni J. *Essentials of Clinical Epilepsy.* Boston: Butterworth-Heinemann; 1999:11–50.

Hauser WA. Seizure disorders: The changes with age. *Epilepsia.* 1992;33: S6–S14.

Holmes GL. Classification of seizures and the epilepsies. In: Schachter SC, Schomer DL, eds. *The Comprehensive Evaluation and Treatment of Epilepsy.* San Diego: Academic Press; 1997:1–36.

Lowenstein DH, Alldredge BK. Status epilepticus at an urban public hospital in the 1980s. *Neurology.* 1993;43:483–488.

Marks WJ, Laxer KD. Semiology of temporal lobe seizures: Value in lateralizing the seizure focus. *Epilepsia*. 1998;39:721–726.

Mizrahi E, Kellaway P. *Diagnosis and Management of Neonatal Seizures*. Philadelphia: Lippincott-Raven; 1998:52.

Morrell MJ. Differential diagnosis of seizures. *Neurol Clin*. 1993;11:737–754.

Murphy JV, Dehkharghani F. Diagnosis of childhood seizure disorders. *Epilepsia*. 1994;35:S7–S17.

Walker M, Shorvon S. Partial epilepsy syndromes in adults. In: Porter RJ, Chadwick D, eds. *The Epilepsies*. Boston: Butterworth-Heinemann; 1997:141–156.

6

Movement Disorders

Matthew D. Troyer

Parkinsonism

Disorder	Distinguishing Features
Parkinson's disease (PD)	Asymmetry of akinesia, rigidity and/or tremor; significant, sustained (>5 years) response to L-dopa. Useful signs when present: classical pill-rolling, parkinsonian rest tremor, and choreiform L-dopa-induced dyskinesias. Absence of early falls, severe autonomic failure, or dementia all favor PD.
Neuroleptic-induced parkinsonism (NIP)	History of neuroleptic or related drug therapy, including metoclopramide; drug withdrawal relieves symptoms but may require weeks or months. Signs and symptoms often symmetrical; more common in women (2:1). Coexisting tardive dyskinesia, akathisia, or rabbit syndrome are highly suggestive of NIP. See *Neuroleptic-Induced Movement Disorders*.
Multiple system atrophy (MSA; striatonigral degeneration, Shy-Drager syndrome, olivopontocerebellar atrophy)	Early and/or severe autonomic symptoms, cerebellar signs, and pyramidal tract signs may coexist with parkinsonism. Dementia occurs rarely. Atypical L-dopa-induced dyskinesias may develop, often in the face. Ancillary studies that may assist diagnosis include autonomic function tests, MRI, and anal sphincter electromyography.
Progressive supranuclear palsy (PSP)	Falls are common early in disease course. Supranuclear palsy of vertical gaze, blepharospasm, axial > limb rigidity/akinesia are distinguishing features. Extended (rather than flexed) posture, pseudobulbar palsy, severe dysarthria and dysphagia also are common; progresses to dementia.
Dementia with Lewy bodies	Dementia is a major feature and may precede, follow, or coexist with parkinsonian signs. Paranoid ideation, florid visual hallucinations, and fluctuating mental state, especially with dopaminergic therapy. Falls are common.
Alzheimer's disease	Dementia is a major, early feature. Parkinsonism may occur in a quarter of Alzheimer's disease patients.
Vascular disease (arteriosclerotic pseudo-parkinsonism, lower-half parkinsonism)	Classically distinguished from PD by a prominent parkinsonian gait without parkinsonian signs in the arms and face ("marche a petits pas"). However, in one series, 3% of patients diagnosed as having PD in life had only lacunar infarcts at autopsy. MRI may be useful.
Normal pressure hydrocephalus	Triad of dementia, incontinence, and a wide-based gait with short steps, reduced step height, and unsteadiness. Often there is a history of past head trauma, meningitis, or subarachnoid hemorrhage.

Parkinsonism is a syndrome defined by the presence of at least two of three cardinal signs: tremor, bradykinesia, and extrapyramidal rigidity. Postural instability also is common. Idiopathic Parkinson's disease is the most common cause of neurodegenerative parkinsonism and is defined by the autopsy findings of Lewy body inclusions and neuronal loss in the substantia nigra. Clinical diagnosis of PD nonetheless can be fairly accurate, although this may be more difficult early in the course of disease. While most PD patients (>95%) respond to L-dopa if an adequate trial is given, individual patients with other causes of parkinsonism also may respond. For example, MSA patients often benefit from L-dopa, but the response typically diminishes within two years.

Quinn (1997); Hughes et al. (1992).

Parkinsonism in Children and Adolescents

Disorder	Age Range	Distinguishing Features
Dopa-responsive dystonia (DRD)	<12 yr	Syndrome of lower limb dystonia with diurnal variation, ± upper limb/axial dystonia. Parkinsonism, including bradykinesia and tremor, may occur. More common in girls. Nonprogressive, very responsive to low-dose L-dopa, and not associated with L-dopa-induced dyskinesias.
Juvenile parkinsonism	Adolescence or early adulthood	Progressive parkinsonism with dystonic features, requiring higher L-dopa doses than DRD. Motor fluctuations and dyskinesias appear early. More common in boys. Some cases are probably a subset of PD; another portion is autosomal recessive juvenile parkinsonism due to mutations in the *parkin* gene on chromosome 6.
Huntington's disease (HD; Westphal variant)	<20	Unlike the choreiform presentation of adult HD, young-onset HD presents as an akinetic-rigid syndrome associated with progressive behavioral changes, dementia, dystonia, and possibly seizures; autosomal dominant.
Wilson's disease	Adolescence or early adulthood	Dystonia, dementia, and prominent tremor. Pure parkinsonism is rare. Also presents with liver disease, Kayser-Fleischer rings.
Hemiparkinsonism-hemiatrophy	Abnormal at birth	Cortical or subcortical atrophy with contralateral parkinsonism and limb atrophy, presumably a result of CNS damage early in life. Variable to good symptomatic response to L-dopa.
Infections or mass lesions involving the basal ganglia	Any	Tumors, viral encephalitis, AIDS, others. Brain imaging and lumbar puncture should be considered for children with parkinsonism without a known genetic etiology.

Jankovic and Fahn (1998).

Dyskinesia

Speed	Characteristics of Movements	Type of Dyskinesia	Associated Disorders
Slowest	Continuous isometric contractions of muscles, even at rest; other features may include prominent truncal involvement with opisthotonos or other abnormal postures, pain, muscle spasms, and abnormal gait	Stiff/rigid syndromes	Stiff person syndrome Neuromyotonia Tetanus
	Nonrhythmic, involuntary, twisting movements and abnormal postures associated with sustained muscle contractions; may be exacerbated by voluntary action and suppressed by sensory tricks (e.g., lightly touching near the affected part)	Dystonia	*See Dystonia* and *Signs of Secondary Dystonia*
	Continuous, rhythmic movements, often complex in nature, including rocking, clapping, hand wringing, and mouthing	Stereotypy	Autism, Schizophrenia Tardive dyskinesia Rett syndrome
	Involuntary, rhythmic oscillations of a body part due to synchronous or alternating muscle contractions	Tremor	*See Rest Tremor, Action Tremor,* and *Parkinson's Disease vs. Essential Tremor*
	Simple or complex, rapid, nonrhythmic movements; the movements are suppressible for a brief period, but this causes a feeling of inner tension relieved by the movement. Movements are exacerbated by stress or anxiety	Tics	Tourette's syndrome Transient tic disorder Drugs/medications (e.g., stimulants such as Ritalin)
	Rapid, often jerky, nonrhythmic, and unpredictable movements that typically flow from one body part to another; usually distal or involving the face	Chorea	*See Chorea in Adults and Chorea in Children and Adolescents*
	Rapid, explosive flinging movements originating proximally in the limbs, generally unilateral	Ballism	*See Chorea in Adults and Chorea in Children and Adolescents*
Fastest	Sudden, nonsuppressible shocklike movements or "jerks"	Myoclonus	*See Myoclonus and Abnormal Facial Movements*

Kishore and Calne (1997).

Chorea in Adults

Etiology	Comments
Huntington's disease (HD)	Progressive disorder that includes behavioral changes, dementia, and dystonia in addition to chorea
Drugs Dopamine receptor blockers L-dopa AEDs Stimulants Oral contraceptives, estrogens Anticholinergics	Dopaminergic blockers are associated with tardive dyskinesia (see *Neuroleptic-Induced Movement Disorders*). L-dopa-induced dyskinesias are common with chronic treatment of PD. AEDs include phenytoin, carbamazepine, and ethosuximide; stimulants include cocaine, amphetamines, methylphenidate, and pemoline.
Endocrine and metabolic causes Chorea gravidarum Hyperthyroidism Hypoglycemia Nonketotic hyperglycemia Electrolyte derangements	Chorea gravidarum may occur in pregnant women with a prior history of Sydenham's chorea, or it may herald SLE or HD. Older women with adult-onset diabetes are most vulnerable to chorea during hyperglycemia; may present as hemichorea. Electrolyte causes include derangements in serum Na, Ca, or Mg.
Infectious diseases	Viral encephalitis, including HIV encephalitis; *Toxoplasma gondii* abscess in AIDS patients; neurosyphilis
Autoimmune disorders	Systemic lupus erythematosus (SLE), antiphospholipid antibody syndrome
Vascular/hematologic disorders Basal ganglia infarction/ischemia Bacterial endocarditis Polycythemia vera	Classically, hemiballism follows subthalamic nucleus infarction, but lesions of other subcortical structures can produce chorea or ballism, which typically resolves in 2–4 weeks.
Idiopathic or genetic disorders Benign essential chorea Senile chorea Spontaneous oral dyskinesia Edentulism Paroxysmal dyskinesias	Benign essential chorea is a nonprogressive, hereditary disorder that begins in childhood. Senile chorea is sporadic, begins after age 60, and consists of generalized chorea. See also *Paroxysmal Movement Disorders*.

Chorea consists of rapid, unpredictable, nonrhythmic movements that flow from one part of the body to another. It can be suppressed transiently by some patients, or it can be incorporated into normal movements. Chorea is often accompanied by motor impersistence, such as difficulty maintaining tongue protrusion or a hand grip. The differential diagnosis of chorea is quite large but most causes are uncommon or rare. Associated signs (e.g., behavioral changes in HD) or clinical setting (e.g., treated PD, pregnancy, renal failure) help narrow the differential.

Mark (1997); Cardoso (1998).

Chorea in Children and Adolescents

Etiology	Comments
Perinatal complications Perinatal asphyxia, kernicterus	Movements begin after age 2; may progress and persist into adulthood. Typically, dystonic movements are also present.
Post-pump (cardiac bypass)	Chorea occurs in infants following cardiac bypass surgery, particularly if hypothermia was used during bypass.

Medications
  Anticonvulsants
  Stimulants
	
	Phenytoin, carbamazepine, and ethosuximide.
	Cocaine, amphetamines including methylphenidate, and pemoline.

Tardive dyskinesia Withdrawal emergent syndrome	See *Neuroleptic-Induced Movement Disorders.* Chorea following abrupt cessation of neuroleptics.

Infectious and postinfectious disorders
  Poststreptococcal (Sydenham's chorea)
  Viral encephalitis
	
	Insidious onset of chorea with emotional lability and hypotonia; usually in school-age children.
	Chorea may be permanent or may resolve spontaneously over several weeks or months.

Endocrine and metabolic causes	Most commonly due to serum Ca, Na, or glucose abnormalities; see also *Chorea in Adults.*

Genetic disorders
  Disorders of amino acid metabolism
  Ataxia-telangiectasia
  Porphyria
  Benign familial chorea
 	
  Paroxysmal dyskinesias
	
	Glutaric aciduria type 1.
	
	A hereditary disorder with onset of chorea in early childhood; may diminish by adolescence.
	See *Paroxysmal Movement Disorders.*

Singer (1998); Cardoso (1998).

Signs of Secondary Dystonia

Parkinsonism	Neuropathy	Supranuclear Oculomotor Palsy	Optic or Retinal Signs	Ataxia
Dopa-responsive dystonia	MLD	Dystonic lipidoses	GM2 gangliosidosis	Ataxia-telangiectasia
Wilson's disease	SCA1 and SCA3	Niemann-Pick type C	NCL	Mitochondrial disorders
Gangliosidosis	Mitochondrial disorders	SCA1 and SCA3	Mitochondrial disorders, including LHON	SCA1 and SCA3
Huntington's disease	Neuroacanthocytosis	Ataxia-telangiectasia	Homocystinuria	MLD
Parkinson's disease		CBGD	Hallervorden-Spatz syndrome	Dystonic lipidoses
PSP		Huntington's disease		NCL
CBGD		Pallidal degeneration		Hartnup's disease
SCA3 (Machado-Joseph)				Wilson's disease
XPD, RPD				
Juvenile Parkinson's disease				
Hallervorden-Spatz syndrome				
Neuroacanthocytosis				
Toxins: Mn, CS$_2$, methanol				
Anoxia				
Hemiparkinsonism-hemiatrophy				
Calcification of basal ganglia				

CBGD: cortical-basal ganglionic degeneration; CS$_2$: carbon disulfide; LHON: Leber's hereditary optic atrophy; MLD: metachromatic leukodystrophy; NCL: neuronal ceroid lipofuscinosis; PSP: progressive supranuclear palsy; RPD: rapid-onset parkinsonism-dystonia; SCA: spinocerebellar atrophy; XPD: X-linked parkinsonism-dystonia.

Dystonia may occur secondary to other disease processes. The associated signs listed here help point to the underlying cause.
Reprinted with permission from Fahn S, Greene PE, Ford B, Bressman SB. *Handbook of Movement Disorders*. Philadelphia: Current Medicine; 1998:64.

Dystonia

	Early Onset (<21 years)	Late Onset (>21 years)
Primary dystonia	Idiopathic torsion dystonia (AD) Other familial dystonias (AD) Sporadic	Sporadic focal/segmental dystonia Task-specific dystonia Familial dystonias (rare, AD)
Dystonia plus	Dopa-responsive dystonia Paroxysmal dyskinesias (see *Paroxysmal Movement Disorders*) Myoclonic dystonia Deficiency of biopterin or enzymes for catecholamine synthesis: tyrosine hydroxylase, aromatic amino acid decarboxylase	
Secondary dystonia	Perinatal cerebral injury Kernicterus Encephalitis, postencephalitic Drugs: neuroleptics, AEDs Stroke and other focal lesions of putamen, thalamus, or midbrain Toxins: Mn, Cu, methanol, cyanide, CO, CS_2, disulfiram, ergot Psychogenic	Stroke and other focal lesions of putamen, thalamus, or midbrain Encephalitis, postencephalitic Drugs: neuroleptics, AEDs Basal ganglia calcification Reflex sympathetic dystrophy Toxins: Mn, Cu, methanol, cyanide, CO, CS_2, disulfiram, ergot Psychogenic
Heredodegenerative diseases	Wilson's disease Juvenile parkinsonism Mitochondrial encephalopathies, such as Leigh's disease Lesch-Nyhan syndrome Disorders of lipid metabolism Organic and amino acid disorders: such as glutaric aciduria type 1 Neuroacanthocytosis Hallervorden-Spatz syndrome	Wilson's disease Machado-Joseph disease (SCA3) Parkinson's disease Parkinson's plus syndromes L-dopa-induced dyskinesias in parkinsonism Dentatorubropallidoluysian atrophy (DRPLA) Neuroacanthocytosis Rapid-onset dystonia-parkinsonism X-linked dystonia-parkinsonism

AD: autosomal dominant; CO: carbon monoxide; CS_2: carbon disulfide.

Dystonia may be divided into early-onset and late-onset groups. Early-onset *primary dystonia* usually starts in an extremity then generalizes to the trunk and other extremities; the causes are mostly hereditary. Late-onset primary dystonia usually starts in the neck, face, or arm muscles and remains focal or segmental. *Dystonia plus* refers to syndromes in which dystonia is accompanied by other movement disorders, such as parkinsonism, chorea, or myoclonus. The differential diagnoses of *secondary dystonia* and *heredodegenerative diseases* associated with dystonia are extensive; only disorders in which dystonia is likely to be a dominant feature are included here.

Jankovic and Fahn (1998); Garcia de Yébenes, Pernaute, Tabernero (1997).

Action Tremor

Causes	Frequency	Activation	Major Features
Physiological tremor, enhanced physiological tremor	6–12 Hz	P, I	8–12 Hz in hands but as slow as 6.5 Hz in other body parts. Tremor frequency decreases with mass loading. Severity is enhanced by anxiety, stress, exercise, fatigue, metabolic derangements, hyperthermia, alcohol withdrawal, and methylxanthines and other stimulants.
Essential tremor (ET)	4–12 Hz	P, K > I	Familial tremor involving the arms (94%), head (33%), voice (12%), and to a lesser degree the legs (16%). Frequency does not change with mass loading. Tremor improves with alcohol in 50–70%. Generally more symmetric than in PD; is slow or nonprogressive. Onset at any age, peak onset at 35–45 yr.
Peripheral neuropathy	3-6 Hz	P > I, K, R	Primarily effects upper extremities; distal tremor frequencies (hand) often slower than proximal (arm); etiologies include HMSN type I, Guillain-Barré syndrome, CIDP, IgG and IgM gammopathies, diabetes, uremia, porphyria.
Dystonic tremor	5-8 Hz	P, I > R	Irregular tremor often affecting the arms or neck in the setting of focal dystonia, e.g., torticollis; improves with a "sensory trick" (e.g., lightly touching the face in torticollis) or by adopting a "null point" posture.
Task-specific tremors			
Primary writing tremor	4–10 Hz	Writing	A form of dystonic tremor.
Isolated voice tremor	3–7 Hz	Speaking	May occur as a focal form of ET or dystonic tremor.
Symptomatic action tremors		P; R, I, P	Medications: valproate, lithium, tricyclic antidepressants, SSRIs. Holmes' tremor (see *Rest Tremor*); Wilson's disease.
Psychogenic tremor	Variable 5–10 Hz	P, I > R	Frequently abrupt in onset with atypical features or mixed frequencies; tremor changes with distraction or suggestion, or frequency may change with contralateral repetitive voluntary movements.
Cerebellar tremor	<4–5 Hz	I > P	Pure or predominantly intention tremor; often unilateral and virtually always symptomatic, e.g., due to MS, trauma, or hereditary ataxias; includes limb tremor, titubation. No rest tremor component. Differential diagnosis includes Holmes' tremor, atypical ET, psychogenic tremor, and Wilson's disease.

R: rest; P: posture holding; K: kinetic; I: intention.

Action tremors are those that occur with muscle activation and may be described as posture holding, kinetic, or intention. For definitions of these terms, see *Rest Tremor*.

Deuschl and Krack (1998).

Rest Tremor

Causes	Tremor Frequency	Activation	Clinical Features
Parkinson's disease	3–6 Hz	R, P	Asymmetric rest tremor present in most PD patients, may involve any limb; "pill rolling" tremor is classic; postural tremor also common (40–60% of patients). Lip or chin tremor may occur.
Neuroleptic-induced parkinsonism	4–6 Hz	R, P	Similar to PD but more often symmetric; nasolabial tremor of rabbit syndrome is a diagnostic clue when present.
Other parkinsonian syndromes	4-6 Hz	R, P	Multisystem atrophy (30–40% of cases); Wilson's disease; less common in PSP. See *Parkinsonism* and *Parkinsonism in Children and Adolescents*.
Holmes tremor (midbrain tremor, rubral tremor)	2–5 Hz, irregular	I, R, P	Jerky, irregular tremor of an arm with prominent proximal involvement; tremor often follows onset of a lesion (e.g., stroke or trauma) involving nigrostriatal and cerebello-thalamic pathways, usually after a delay of weeks to months. Ataxia, pyramidal weakness, CN III involvement or dystonia also may be present.

R: rest tremor, occurs in a body part at rest, with no voluntary muscle activation; P: tremor occurs during posture holding, such as holding arms away from body; I: intention tremor, occurs at the end of a goal-directed movement; K: kinetic tremor, occurs during movement of a limb.

Deuschl and Krack (1998).

Parkinson's Disease vs. Essential Tremor

	Parkinson's Disease	*Essential Tremor*
Tremor	Occurs at rest, decreases with action, may resume with posture holding; increases while walking	Occurs with posture holding and action
Distribution	Asymmetrical, sometimes unilateral	Relatively symmetrical
Body part	Hands, legs	Hands, head, voice
Drawing a spiral	Micrographic	Tremulous
Age at onset	Middle age or later (mean = 59 yr)	All ages (mean = 35–45 yr)
Course	Progressive	Stable or slowly progressive
First-degree relatives	Usually unaffected	Often affected
Other neurologic signs	Bradykinesia, rigidity, postural instability	None
Agents that decrease tremor	Anticholinergics, L-dopa, dopamine agonists	Alcohol, propranolol, primidone, benzodiazepines

One of the most common misdiagnoses in neurology is mistaking essential tremor for Parkinson's disease. The presence of resting tremor, associated rigidity and bradykinesia, and response to L-dopa should distinguish PD from the symptomatology of ET.

Modified with permission from Fahn S, Greene PE, Ford B, Bressman SB. *Handbook of Movement Disorders*. Philadelphia: Current Medicine; 1998.

Myoclonus

Presentation	Disorders	Clinical Features and Causes
Myoclonus occurring in isolation	Physiological myoclonus	Myoclonus occurs in specific circumstances, including sleep (hypnic) jerks, hiccups, and benign infantile myoclonus with feeding; absence of other neurologic signs
Generalized or multifocal myoclonus with no evidence of encephalopathy	Essential myoclonus	Onset before age 20, benign course; often improves with ethanol consumption; sporadic or AD inheritance
	Myoclonic dystonia (dystonia-myoclonus syndrome)	Dystonia and myoclonic jerks mostly affecting the neck, trunk, and arms; AD; improves with ethanol
Generalized or multifocal myoclonus with or without encephalopathy	Toxic or metabolic encephalopathy	Renal or hepatic failure; medications, drugs, or toxins, including anticonvulsants, serotonergic agents (trazodone, tricyclics), serotonin syndrome, clozapine, dopaminergic agents, lead
	Postanoxic myoclonus (Lance-Adams syndrome)	Action myoclonus following coma due to cardiopulmonary arrest; ataxia also is common
Epileptic myoclonus	Infantile myoclonus	Clinical syndromes dominated by seizures without progressive encephalopathy; see *Myoclonic Seizures in Infants*, in Chapter 5
	Lennox-Gastaut syndrome	
	Myoclonic absences in petit mal epilepsy	
	EPC	
	Juvenile myoclonic epilepsy	
Progressive myoclonic epilepsy	See *Progressive Myoclonus Epilepsy*, in Chapter 5	Clinical epilepsy syndromes with progressive encephalopathy as a dominant feature
Spinal segmental myoclonus	Focal cord lesions, most commonly trauma or tumor but also other mass lesions, vascular causes, and MS	Repetitive, often rhythmic contractions of muscles innervated by one or a few adjacent spinal levels
Focal myoclonus	Focal lesions, often involving the cortex, including stroke, trauma, tumor; focal seizures (EPC)	Focal, sometimes rhythmic myoclonic jerks that may be induced by sensory stimulation or action

EPC: epilepsia partialis continua.

Obeso (1997); Fahn et al. (1998).

130

Neuroleptic-Induced Movement Disorders

Movement Disorder	Time Course	Features
Acute dystonic reaction	Immediate to days after starting agent	Abnormal sustained muscle contractions or postures; may affect neck, face, tongue, eyes (oculogyric crisis), trunk, and limbs
Acute akathisia	Immediate or acute	Inability to sit or stand still; patient feels a sense of inner restlessness
Neuroleptic-induced parkinsonism	Subacute, insidious	Dose-related parkinsonism in which all cardinal signs of PD may occur; may coexist with "rabbit syndrome" or TD
Withdrawal emergent syndrome	Occurs following abrupt withdrawal from chronic neuroleptic therapy	Generalized choreic movements involving trunk, limbs, neck, and rarely the face; usually occurs in children
Neuroleptic malignant syndrome	Begins abruptly while on neuroleptic therapy or after rapid withdrawal of dopaminergic agents	Muscle rigidity with elevated CPK, fever, autonomic hyperactivity, and alteration of mental status
Classical TD	Chronic, late, and persistent	Repetitive, chorea-like oro-buccolingual chewing movements; limb chorea often present
Tardive dystonia	Chronic, late, and persistent	Sustained involuntary torsional movements of neck, trunk, oral region, or face; limb chorea also may occur
Tardive akathisia	Chronic, late, and persistent	Sensation of inner restlessness and intolerance of remaining still, with overt movements of restlessness, pacing, marching in place, and fidgetiness

TD: tardive dyskinesia.

Tardive syndromes are abnormal involuntary movements caused by exposure to dopamine receptor blocking agents that persist for at least 1 month after withdrawal of the drug. The risk of developing a tardive syndrome increases with duration of exposure and is greater with older, high-potency agents (e.g., haloperidol) than with newer drugs (risperidone, clozapine).

Modified with permission from Fahn S, Greene PE, Ford B, Bressman SB. *Handbook of Movement Disorders*. Philadelphia: Current Medicine; 1998.

Abnormal Facial Movements

Movement Disorder	Age	Side	Control	Sleep	Clinical Characteristics	Associations
Blepharospasm	>50	Bilateral	Some	No	Bilateral synchronous spasms of orbicularis oculi	Essential blepharospasm, Meige's syndrome, PSP, midbrain or thalamic lesions
Oromandibular dystonia	Any	Bilateral	No	No	Prolonged dystonic movements, often with blepharospasm and involvement of forehead, oromandibular muscles, and platysma; no limb dyskinesias	Meige's syndrome, acute dystonic reaction, tardive dystonia, midbrain or thalamic lesions, Wilson's disease
Tardive dyskinesia	Any	Bilateral	Yes	No	Choreiform and stereotyped movements of lower face including chewing, grimacing, tongue protrusion	Neuroleptic medications; similar dyskinesias occur in edentulism and buccal-oral-lingual dyskinesia of aging
Essential tremor	Any	Bilateral	No	No	Tremor may affect facial muscles, voice, head, and limbs	Probably a genetic disorder, autosomal dominant with incomplete penetrance
Rabbit syndrome	Any	Bilateral	No	No	Rabbitlike 3–6 Hz vertical tremor of perioral and perinasal muscles	Neuroleptic medications, NIP
Facial tics	Onset <20	Uni- or bilateral	Yes	Yes	Stereotypic movements: rapid, brief, repetitive; suppressible	Tourette's syndrome or idiopathic
Hemifacial spasm	50–70	Unilateral	No	±	Tonic or clonic movements of muscles innervated by CN VII	Microvascular compression of CN VII, tumor, aneurysm, AVM, MS or stroke
Facial synkinesis	Any	Unilateral	No	Yes	Unilateral facial weakness; abnormal movements occur with voluntary movements of the involved side	Prior history of Bell's palsy, surgery or trauma to CN VII
Myokymia	Any	Unilateral	No	Yes	Constant, rapid undulating and flickering muscles; "bag of worms"	MS, brainstem tumor

NIP: neuroleptic-induced parkinsonism.

Control: Does patient have voluntary control of movement? Sleep: Is movement present in sleep?

Modified with permission from Digre K, Corbett JJ. Hemifacial spasm: Differential diagnosis, mechanism, and treatment. In: Jankovic J, Tolosa E, eds. *Facial Dyskinesias*. Vol. 49. New York: Raven Press; 1988.

Paroxysmal Movement Disorders

	PKC	PED	PDC	PND	EA1	EA2
Age at onset (yr)	1–40	2–20	1–30	10–40	2–15	5–15
Duration	Brief (<5 min)	Intermediate (5–30 min)	Prolonged (2 min–4 hr)	Short: <1 min; long: 5–30 min	2–10 min	Can last many hours or days
Frequency	Up to 100/day	2/month–1/day	2/year–3/day	2/year–5/night	Up to 15/day	<1/month–daily
Triggers	Sudden movement, startle	Prolonged exercise or cold	Fatigue, caffeine, alcohol	Primarily during non-REM sleep	Sudden movement, startle	Stress, fatigue, alcohol, caffeine
Features of the attacks	Dystonia + chorea unilateral, alternating or bilateral	Dystonia ± chorea, prominent leg involvement	Dystonia ± chorea	Dystonic posturing and jerking movements	Ataxia, weakness, dysarthria, tremor, facial twitching	Ataxia, dysarthria, vertigo, diplopia, weakness
Other neurologic features	Normal between attacks	Normal between attacks	Normal between attacks	Rare daytime attacks; tonic-clonic seizures also may occur	Interictal myokymia and neuromyotonia with no ataxia	Gaze-evoked nystagmus and mild ataxia
Etiology	AD or sporadic	AD	AD with linkage to chromosome 2q or sporadic	Short attacks: sporadic or AD vs. medial frontal lobe epilepsy	AD with linkage to K+ channel gene KCNA1 on chromosome 12p	AD with mutations in calcium channel gene CACNA1A at 19p13
Effective treatments	Carbamazepine other AEDs, acetazolamide	None except avoiding prolonged exercise	Limited response to benzodiazepines; avoid precipitants	Short attacks: AEDs; Long: acetazolamide, haloperidol	Acetazolamide, phenytoin	Acetazolamide

PKC: paroxysmal kinesogenic choreoathetosis; PED: paroxysmal exercise-induced dystonia; PDC: paroxysmal dystonic (nonkinesogenic) choreoathetosis; PND: paroxysmal nocturnal dyskinesia; EA1: episodic ataxia with myokymia; EA2: episodic ataxia with no myokymia.

Paroxysmal choreoathetosis, or paroxysmal dyskinesias, are episodic movement disorders best diagnosed by history, since the patients show no abnormal features between attacks. This group of disorders classically is divided into PKC, PED, and PDC, based on clinical features. PND probably is a heterogeneous condition, with short attacks arising from frontal lobe seizures and longer attacks due to a movement disorder. These disorders and the episodic ataxias may result from mutations in ion channel proteins.

Sethi (1998); Massaquoi and Hallett (1998).

REFERENCES

Cardoso F. Infectious and transmissible movement disorders. In: Jankovic J, Tolosa E, eds. *Parkinson's Disease and Movement Disorders*. Baltimore: Williams & Wilkins; 1998:945–965.

Deuschl G, Krack P. Tremors: Differential diagnosis, neurophysiology and pharmacology. In: Jankovic J, Tolosa E, eds. *Parkinson's Disease and Movement Disorders*. Baltimore: Williams & Wilkins; 1998:419–452.

Digre K, Corbett JJ. Hemifacial spasm: Differential diagnosis, mechanism, and treatment. In: Jankovic J, Tolosa E, eds. *Facial Dyskinesias*. Vol. 49. New York: Raven Press: 1988:151–176.

Fahn S, Greene PE, Ford B, Bressman SB. *Handbook of Movement Disorders*. Philadelphia: Current Medicine; 1998.

Garcia de Yébenes J, Pernaute RS, Tabernero C. Symptomatic dystonias. In: Watts RL, Koller WC, eds. *Movement Disorders: Neurologic Principles and Practice*. New York: McGraw-Hill; 1997:455–475.

Hughes AJ, Daniel SE, Kilford L, Lees AJ. Accuracy of clinical diagnosis of idiopathic Parkinson's disease: A clinico-pathological study of 100 cases. *J Neurol Neurosurg Psych*. 1992;55:181–184.

Jankovic J, Fahn S. Dystonic disorders. In: Jankovic J, Tolosa E, eds. *Parkinson's Disease and Movement Disorders*. Baltimore: Williams & Wilkins; 1998:513–551.

Kishore A, Calne DB. Approach to the patient with a movement disorder and overview of movement disorders. In: Watts RL, Koller WC, eds. *Movement Disorders: Neurologic Principles and Practice*. New York: McGraw-Hill; 1997:3–14.

Mark MH. Other choreatic disorders. In: Watts RL, Koller WC, eds. *Movement Disorders: Neurologic Principles and Practice*. New York: McGraw-Hill; 1997:527–539.

Massaquoi SG, Hallett M. Ataxia and other cerebellar syndromes. In: Jankovic J, Tolosa E, eds. *Parkinson's Disease and Movement Disorders*. Baltimore: Williams & Wilkins; 1998:632–686.

Obeso JA. Classification, clinical features, and treatment of myoclonus. In: Watts RL, Koller WC, eds. *Movement Disorders: Neurologic Principles and Practice*. New York: McGraw-Hill; 1997:541–550.

Quinn NP, ed. *Parkinsonism*. Baillière's Clinical Neurology. Vol. 6. London: Baillière Tindall; 1997.

Sethi KD. Paroxysmal dyskinesias. In: Jankovic J, Tolosa E, eds. *Parkinson's Disease and Movement Disorders*. Baltimore: Williams & Wilkins; 1998: 701–708.

Singer HS. Movement disorders in children. In: Jankovic J, Tolosa E, eds. *Parkinson's Disease and Movement Disorders*. Baltimore: Williams & Wilkins; 1998:729–753.

7

Degenerative Disorders

Ericka P. Simpson

Acquired Motor Neuron Diseases

Disease	Clinical Features
Amyotrophic lateral sclerosis (ALS)	Progressive pure motor disorder, with diffuse lower and upper motor neuron signs. Due to loss of motor neurons in the anterior spinal cord, brainstem, and motor cortex. Most common motor neuron disease.
Primary lateral sclerosis (PLS)	Slow, progressive upper motor neuron disorder that begins with symmetric, spastic paraparesis due to involvement of corticospinal tracts. Diagnosis requires exclusion of other causes of spastic paraparesis (e.g., MS, adrenoleukodystrophy, spinal cord lesions).
Progressive bulbar palsy/ progressive muscular atrophy	Lower motor neuron involvement only (weakness, muscle atrophy, and hypo- or areflexia) of bulbar and skeletal muscles. There is clinical overlap with ALS, and some cases that initially have only LMN findings may evolve into ALS.
Poliomyelitis	Acute destruction of lower motor neurons by any of the polio enteroviruses that infect the GI tract. Presents as a mild flulike illness with fever, meningismus, and headache followed by weakness of striated muscles. Nearly eradicated in countries with vaccination programs.
Postpolio syndrome/ progressive postpolio muscular atrophy (PPMA)	New, progressive weakness and muscle atrophy occurring 10–30 years after recovery from the acute polio infection. New weakness often involves both previously affected muscles and unaffected muscles.
Echovirus, coxsackie, enterovirus	Other viruses may cause a paralytic illness resembling poliomyelitis but also may involve other organs, such as the heart as in the case of coxsackie.
Hyperparathyroidism/ hyperthyroidism	May produce an ALS-like syndrome with rare cases showing reversal of symptoms with treatment of the endocrinopathy
Lead or mercury intoxication	Can cause an ALS-like syndrome. There usually is a definite history of exposure. Some patients show improvement with chelating therapy or withdrawal of toxin.
Paraproteinemia/ lymphoma	There are reports of an association between lymphoma and ALS. Some of these patients may be diagnosed by the presence of a monoclonal gammopathy or an increase in CSF protein.

LMN: lower motor neuron.

Brooks (1996); Ross (1997).

Signs and Symptoms of Amyotrophic Lateral Sclerosis

Motor System	Signs and Symptoms
Lower motor neuron	Weakness Muscle atrophy, cramps, fasciculations Hyporeflexia, areflexia
Upper motor neuron	Weakness, spasticity, loss of dexterity Pseudobulbar affect Hyperreflexia
Upper and lower motor neuron	Dysarthria Dysphagia Respiratory dysfunction
Atypical	Sensory dysfunction or pain Autonomic dysfunction Bowel/bladder dysfunction Dementia Oculomotor dysfunction

Amyotrophic lateral sclerosis (ALS; Lou Gehrig's disease) is the most common of motor neuron disorders. Of all cases, 90–95% are sporadic; of the familial cases, about 20% are due to a defect in the gene for the copper-zinc superoxide dismutase enzyme (SOD1). The overall incidence is 1–2:100,000 worldwide and increases with age. The disease occurs primarily in adult life, with a slight male predominance. Interestingly, oculomotor and bowel and bladder dysfunction are not clinically apparent in ALS patients until late in the disease. ALS is a progressive disease that results in death within 3 years in 50% of patients, usually due to respiratory failure. While there is no known cure for the disease, riluzole, a glutamate receptor antagonist, has been shown to delay the rate of progression by about 10%.

Jackson and Bryan (1998).

Diagnosis of Amyotrophic Lateral Sclerosis

Suspected	Lower motor neuron findings in at least two regions No upper motor neuron dysfunction
Possible	Upper motor and lower motor neuron findings in one region, or upper motor neuron findings in at least two regions
Probable	Upper motor neuron findings in at least two regions, and lower motor neuron findings in at least two regions, and at least one upper motor neuron finding rostral to at least one lower motor neuron finding
Definite	Upper motor neuron and lower motor neuron findings in at least three out of four regions
Proven	Confirmation of clinical presentation by postmortem examination

ALS ultimately is a clinical diagnosis and depends on findings of lower and upper motor neuron disease in multiple regions, as well as exclusion of other, potentially treatable diseases. An initially tentative diagnosis may become more secure as the disease progresses; therefore, clinical reevaluation is necessary. And, because the prognosis is grave, the diagnosis should be confirmed by at least two physicians. The categories here represent the *El Escorial* criteria, which were revised in 1998 to include preclinical lower motor neuron signs in a region other than that found on physical exam; this requires EMG documentation of denervation in at least two muscles of different root and nerve origin in two different limbs. *Regions* are defined here as bulbar, cervical, thoracic, or lumbosacral. Laboratory and electrophysiology studies that should be considered when evaluating a potential case of ALS include (and this is not an exhaustive list):

Routine labs	ESR, CK, SPEP, parathyroid hormone, TFTs, B_{12}, CBC, serum chemistries.
Electrophysiology	EMG: spontaneous activity in affected muscles at rest—positive sharp waves, fasciculations, fibrillations. NCS: Usually normal with exception of decreased CMAP due to motor neuron death.
Radiography	MRI or CT of brain ± cervical cord to rule out other pathology. In typical ALS, scans usually are normal except for degeneration of corticospinal tracts.
Other	Muscle biopsy not necessary in most cases. Useful if there is suspicion of myopathy or minimal motor neuron involvement is evident.

CMAP: compound muscle action potential.

Brooks (1999); Jackson and Bryan (1998); Rowland (1998).

Atypical Features of Amyotrophic Lateral Sclerosis

Atypical Feature	*Alternative Diagnoses*
Sensory dysfunction	Polyneuropathy (multiple etiologies, including mononeuritis multiplex) Chronic inflammatory demyelinating polyneuropathy (CIDP) Vitamin B_{12} deficiency Hereditary spastic paraparesis, multiple sclerosis, spinal cord pathology (compression, invasion, ischemia, radiation)
Dementia	ALS-Parkinson-dementia complex (Guamanian complex), frontal lobe dementia, prion disease (e.g., Creutzfeld-Jakob disease), lead or mercury poisoning, hypothyroidism, hyperparathyroidism, B_{12} deficiency
Oculomotor dysfunction	Cranial or spinal radiculopathy (e.g., Lyme disease, CMV), cranial or peripheral neuropathy (diabetes; toxicity from dapsone, INH, lead, or mercury)
Symmetric, proximal weakness	Myopathy, polymyositis, limb-girdle muscular dystrophy, spinal muscular atrophy, Lambert-Eaton myasthenic syndrome
Symmetric, distal weakness	Inclusion body myositis, polyneuropathy
No bulbar involvement	Spinal cord pathology: cervical spondylitic myelopathy, tumor, disc herniation, postradiation, arteriovenous malformation, syrinx
Bowel or bladder dysfunction	Spinal cord pathology, multiple sclerosis
Age <30 yr	Hexosaminidase A deficiency
Only upper motor neuron signs and symptoms	Hereditary or tropical spastic paraparesis, multiple sclerosis, primary lateral sclerosis, lower brainstem or spinal cord pathology
Pure lower motor neuron	Spinal muscular atrophy, Kennedy's syndrome, multifocal motor neuropathy, progressive muscular atrophy, poliomyelitis, post-polio syndrome, hexosaminidase A deficiency, polyneuropathy
Significant weight loss, anorexia, general wasting, and cachexia	Neoplasm (lymphoma, leukemia), paraneoplastic syndrome, HIV-associated myelopathy

Cole and Siddique (1999); Jackson and Bryan (1998); Ross (1997).

Diseases That Mimic Amyotrophic Lateral Sclerosis

	Amyotrophic Lateral Sclerosis (ALS)	Multifocal Motor Neuropathy (MMN)	Chronic Inflammatory Demyelinating Polyneuropathy (CIDP)	Inclusion Body Myositis (IBM)
Incidence	1–2:100,000	Unknown, rare	10–20% of all undiagnosed neuropathies	Most common myopathy >55 yr of age
M:F ratio	1.5–2:1	4:1	1.5:1	Male predominance
Age of onset (yr)	50–60 (peaks at 75)	20–50 (average 41)	All ages (peaks 40–60)	50–70 (mean 63)
Clinical features	Progressive asymmetric weakness. Bulbar and respiratory involvement. No sensory involvement. Fasciculations in clinically normal and involved muscles.	Progressive asymmetric weakness. Bulbar and respiratory involvement rare. No sensory involvement. Fasciculations in clinically involved muscles only.	Progressive symmetric stepwise or relapsing weakness ≥2 mo. Bulbar, respiratory, or autonomic involvement uncommon. Sensory involvement common. Fasciculations rare.	Insidious symmetric muscle weakness with predominant weakness of quadriceps femoris and forearm muscles (especially finger flexors). Bulbar weakness causing dysphagia in 20–30%.
Lab findings	CSF: normal. CK: mildly ↑ or normal. 50% have low titers of anti-GM1 antibodies.	CSF: nl (>90%). CK: mild–moderate ↑ or normal. 50–85% have IgM-GM1 ± IgM-asialo-GM1 or GM2 antibodies.	CSF: 94% have protein >45 and cell count <10.	CSF: normal. CK: normal or mildly ↑
NCS/EMG	NCS: normal except for decreased CMAP. EMG: neurogenic pattern with denervation/reinnervation pattern in clinically weakened and normal muscles.	NCS: complete or partial motor conduction block outside usual sites of compression. Normal SNAP at sites of conduction block. EMG: neurogenic pattern confined to muscles innervated by nerves with block.	NCS: slowed motor and sensory velocities in ≥2 nerves. Conduction block or temporal dispersion ≥1 nerve. Absent or prolonged F waves. EMG: symmetric neurogenic pattern in distribution of nerve involvement.	NCS: ± motor conduction velocities reduced and sensory latencies prolonged. EMG: myopathic pattern ± a neurogenic pattern in a minority of patients.

CMAP: compound muscle action potential; SNAP: sensory nerve action potential.

See also *Multifocal Motor Neuropathy*, in Chapter 9.

Bentes et al. (1999); Bouche et al. (1999); Chaudhry (1998),

Inherited Motor Neuron Disorders

Disorder	Inheritance	Chromosome	Clinical Features
Spinal muscular atrophies (SMAs)	AR	5q11.2–13.3	LMN
Amyotrophic lateral sclerosis (ALS)	AD	21q22.1 (2% of ALS cases)	LMN and UMN
Juvenile onset amyotrophic lateral sclerosis	AD	9q34	UMN and LMN No bulbar involvement
	AR type I	15q5–q22	LMN > UMN
	AR type II	Unknown	LMN and UMN (legs only)
	AR type III	2q33	UMN > LMN
Kennedy disease	XLR	Xq21–22	LMN Testicular atrophy, glucose intolerance, gynecomastia
Hereditary spastic paraplegia	AD, AR, X-linked	12 different loci identified	UMN ± extrapyramidal signs, dementia, ataxia, icthyosis, deafness, optic neuropathy

LMN: lower motor neuron weakness; UMN: upper motor neuron weakness.

With the exception of the spinal muscular atrophies, inherited motor neuron disease is relatively rare. For example, only ~5% of ALS is inherited; of this, about 20–25% of cases have been associated with mutations in the cytoplasmic superoxide dismutase enzyme. While juvenile ALS is even more rare, it has a penetrance of 100% by 20 years of age.

Note that Kennedy disease is unique among inherited motor neuron diseases for being a triplet repeat disease: Clinical disease is associated with an increase in CAG nucleotide repeats (>347) encoding a polyglutamine stretch within the first exon of the androgen receptor gene.

See also *Spinal Muscular Atrophy*.

Modified with permission from Cole N, Siddique T. Genetic disorders of motor neurons. *Semin Neurol.* 1999.

Spinal Muscular Atrophy

Type	Inheritance	Symptom Onset	Clinical Features	Prognosis
SMA I (Werdnig-Hoffmann disease)	AR XLR (rare)	Birth–6 mo. Decreased fetal movements may be apparent	Hypotonia, weakness. Problems with suck, swallowing, breathing	95% dead <1 yr (average 8 mo.)
SMA II	AR	3–15 mo.	Proximal lower extremity weakness, fasciculations, fine hand tremor	Median survival 12 yr
SMA III (Kugelberg-Welander disease)	AR, AD	5–15 yr	Proximal lower extremity weakness, delayed motor milestones	Survival into adulthood, but wheelchair bound in 30s.
SMA IV	AR, AD	Adulthood (average 37 yr)	Proximal weakness, variable and more severe in AD form	Life expectancy near normal
Distal SMA	AD, AR	AR: birth or infancy AD: adulthood	Distal weakness	Slow clinical course Life expectancy normal

Spinal muscular atrophy (SMA) is a set of inherited neurodegenerative disorders characterized by loss of spinal and bulbar motor neurons, resulting in muscle weakness and atrophy. The incidence is 1:10,000 newborns, and it is the most frequent fatal autosomal disorder among infants. The inheritance is mostly autosomal recessive, but there are X-linked and autosomal dominant forms. There are four types of SMA, with the worst clinical severity observed in type I. The gene loci for the three early forms have been mapped to a region on chromosome 5q11.2–13.3, which encodes for four genes: *SMN1*, *SMN2*, *NAIP*, and *H4F5*. The most important of these is the novel protein, survival motor neuron (SMN), which influences mRNA metabolism.

No specific therapy exists for any of the SMAs. Management is aimed at preventing respiratory complications, poor nutrition, skeletal deformities, and social isolation.

Modified with permission from Cole N, Siddique T. Genetic disorders of motor neurons. *Semin Neurol.* 1999.

Biros and Forrest (1999).

Neurodegenerative Movement Disorders with Dementia

Disease	Onset (yr)/Incidence	Clinical Features
Parkinson's disease	40–70; peaks in 50s M:F = 1:1 30–300:100,000 prevalence in those >40	30% have a predominantly subcortical dementia that follows development of PD signs and symptoms (rigidity, bradykinesia, resting tremor, postural instability)
Dementia with Lewy bodies	50–80 (average 72) M:F = 2:1 Second commonest diagnosis of dementia	Fluctuating dementia, psychosis with florid hallucinations, and extrapyramidal signs and symptoms (rigidity, bradykinesia)
Progressive supranuclear palsy	50–70 5:100,000	Gait disturbance with early falls, axial > limb rigidity, impaired vertical (especially downward) gaze, dysarthria/dysphagia, and subcortical dementia
Huntington's disease	30–50 M > F 5–9:100,000 prevalence	Personality and behavior changes, dementia, chorea AD inheritance (Chr. 4) Death within 15 years of onset Westphal variant: rapidly progressive childhood form with akinetic-rigid syndrome, mental retardation, seizures
Wilson's disease	Adolescence to early adulthood 3:100,000 prevalence	Psychiatric symptoms and variable dementia, akinetic-rigid syndrome, "wing-beating" tremor with hepatic dysfunction, decreased serum ceruloplasmin levels AR inheritance (Chr. 13)
Creutzfeldt-Jakob disease	35–65 1:1,000,000	Cognitive decline, myoclonus, cerebellar signs, pyramidal signs, parkinsonism
ALS-Parkinson-dementia complex of Guam	Middle-late adulthood (average 57) in Chamarro Indians M > F	Combination of symptoms characteristic of parkinsonism, dementia, and motor neuron disease ± supranuclear palsy Death occurs in ~5 years after onset
Hallervorden-Spatz disease	First two decades Rare	Presents with parkinsonism, dystonia, dementia, disturbances in speech and gait AR inheritance (Chr. 20)

See also *Parkinsonism*, in Chapter 6.

Perkin (1997); Rodnitzky (1999).

Early-Onset Dementia

Disease	Clinical Features
Familial Alzheimer's dementia	Most early-onset Alzheimer's disease (<65 yr) is familial, with AD inheritance Associated with amyloid precursor protein (APP) gene mutations on Chr. 21, presenilin 1 mutations on Chr. 14, and presenilin 2 mutations on Chr. 1
Huntington's disease	AD inheritance (Chr. 4) Chorea, psychiatric symptoms, and dementia Typical onset is in 30s and progresses over 15–20 yr; onset <20 yr termed *Westphal variant*
Wilson's disease	AR inherited mutation on Chr. 13 Cognitive decline progressing to frank dementia, associated with psychiatric symptoms, movement disorders, and hepatic dysfunction Mean onset 21 yr, equally divided among neurologic, psychiatric, and hepatic presentations
Adult neuronal ceroid lipofuscinosis (Kuf's disease)	AR or AD inheritance Onset in adolescence to middle age adulthood Seizures, dementia, ataxia See also *Progressive Myoclonus Epilepsy*, in Chapter 5.
Adult-onset metachromatic leukodystrophy (MLD)	AR inheritance due to deficiency of arylsulfatase A Often presents with psychiatric illness or dementia, ataxia, spasticity, speech defects Course is prolonged and survival into the 40s or 50s is possible
Creutzfeldt-Jakob disease	Most common of spongiform encephalopathies and occurs in sporadic, inherited, or transmitted forms Peak age of onset is 55–75 yr (mean 61 yr); familial form has AD inheritance and average onset of 55 yr; "new variant" CJD emerged (1994–1995) in the United Kingdom, with an average age of onset of 28 yr Rapidly progressive dementia, myoclonus, visual abnormalities, cerebellar dysfunction, gait and speech abnormalities EEG with periodic triphasic sharp waves
Gerstmann-Sträussler-Scheinker syndrome	AD inherited prion disease Dementia, cerebellar signs, gait and speech abnormalities Age of onset in 40–50s
Fatal familial insomnia	AD inherited prion disease Progressive insomnia, autonomic dysfunction, severe dementia Average age of onset 49.3 (range 25–72 yr)
HIV-associated dementia	Develops in 15–20% of cases with advanced disease Leading cause of dementia in the young Progressive psychomotor slowing, memory impairment

See also *Neurodegenerative Causes of Dementia,* in Chapter 11.

Belay (1999); Geyer, Keating, Potts (1998); Liang (1998); McArthur, Sacktor, Selnes (1999).

146

Mitochondrial Disorders

	MERFF	MELAS	KSS	NARP
Syndromic features				
Seizures	•	+		
Ataxia	•	+	+	•
Myoclonus	•	±		
Hemiparesis/hemianopsia		•		
Cortical blindness		•		
Migrainous headache		•		
Ophthalmoplegia			•	
Pigmentary retinopathy			•	
Cardiac conduction block		±	•	
Peripheral neuropathy	+	+	+	•
Nonsyndromic features				
Weakness	+	+	+	+
Short stature	+	+	+	
Deafness	+	+		±
Dementia/regression	±	+	+	
Lactic acidosis	+	+	+	
Ragged red fibers	+	+	+	
Maternal inheritance	+	+		+
Sporadic inheritance			+	

+: usually present; ±: often present; •: required for diagnosis: MERRF: myoclonus epilepsy with ragged red fibers; MELAS: mitochondrial encephalomyopathy, lactic acidosis, and strokelike episodes; KSS: Kearns-Sayre syndrome: NARP: neuropathy, ataxia, and retinitis pigmentosa.

Mitochondrial disorders are a set of diseases resulting from mutations or deletions in the mitochondrial genome. Their presentation comprises a spectrum of signs and symptoms, some of which are syndromic (that is, tend to appear together to define a single syndrome) and others of which are common to a number of mitochondrial syndromes. It is increasingly appreciated that mitochondrial disease may present with single "nonsyndromic" signs and symptoms, such as isolated deafness. This list contains the more frequent manifestations of mitochondrial disease and is not exhaustive. Another mitochondrial disease not listed here is Leber's hereditary optic neuropathy (LHON), with blindness, psychiatric symptoms, ataxia, and peripheral neuropathy.

Dimauro and Bonilla (1997); DiMauro and Schon (1998).

Degenerative Disease Caused by Nutritional Deficiency

Vitamin Deficiency and Causes	Clinical Features	Mechanism
Vitamin B_{12}		
Decreased or no intrinsic factor production by parietal cells (due to pernicious anemia, gastrectomy) Ileal malabsorption, strict vegetarianism, drugs	Dementia, encephalopathy Sensory neuropathy Myelopathy (subacute combined degeneration) Visual impairment	Methionine synthesis is impaired due to inability to transfer methyl groups to methionine. Interferes with protein and polyamine synthesis
Folate		
Coexists with alcoholism, generalized malabsorption, anticonvulsant therapy	Subacute combined deficiency-like syndrome, dementia, neuropathy, vasculopathy (causing stroke), neural tube defects	Folic acid derivative, methyltetrahydrofolate, central to vitamin B_{12}-dependent reaction that converts homocysteine to methionine
Vitamin E		
Fat malabsorption syndromes (enterohepatic dysfunction, cystic fibrosis, Bassen-Kornzweig syndrome)	Weakness or gait incoordination Spinocerebellar degeneration ± peripheral nerve involvement yielding ataxia and areflexia	Scavenger of free radicals Fat-soluble and dependent on bile salts for absorption in small intestine
Nicotinic acid		
Dietary deficiency, corn-heavy diet	Pellagra: diarrhea, dementia, dermatitis	Converted to two important coenzymes in carbohydrate metabolism: NAD, NADPH.
Vitamin B_6 (pyridoxine)		
Pyridoxine-deficient breast milk, congenital pyridoxine deficiency Drugs: INH, hydralazine, penicillamine	Infantile spasms INH-related polyneuropathy in slow inactivators	Pyroxidal phosphate is a coenzyme important for metabolism of many amino acids
Thiamine		
Alcohol abuse Rice-heavy diets	Wernicke-Korsakoff syndrome Beriberi polyneuropathy and cardiomyopathy	Precursor for coenzyme thiamine pyrophosphate; catalyzes the oxidative decarboxylation of pyruvate, α-ketoglutarate, and eventually coenzyme A

Vitamin D		
Malabsorption syndromes	Myopathic weakness in the pelvic girdle and neck muscles causing a waddling gait	Calcium, phosphate homeostasis; pathogenic mechanism in muscle is obscure
Anticonvulsants		
Dietary deficiency	Osteomalacia	
Vitamin A		
Malabsorption syndromes	Reduced night vision	Aldehyde form, retinal, forms rhodopsin, which is responsible for night vision
	Keratinization of conjunctiva and cornea	

So and Simon (2000).

Inherited Causes of Degenerative Ataxia

Disease	Age of Onset/Course	Inheritance/ Chromosome	Clinical Features
Friedreich's ataxia	Onset usually 8–15 yr; wheelchair-bound 15 yr after onset; average survival into 30s 1:20,000 incidence	AR/9q	Gait and limb ataxia, dysarthria, areflexia, sensory loss, pyramidal tract disease, cardiomyopathy, skeletal deformities, diabetes or impaired glucose tolerance Most common AR inherited ataxia
Ataxia with isolated vitamin E deficiency	Begins in childhood or adolescence	AR/ 8q13 Gene for α-tocopherol transfer protein	FA-like phenotype
Ataxia-telangiectasia	Onset in first year Survival into 20s 1:80,000 incidence	AR/11q ATM gene responsible for DNA repair	Progressive ataxia, oculocutaneous telangiectasia, choreoathetosis, dystonia, distal muscle atrophy, predisposition to recurrent infection and malignancy (lymphoma)
SCA1 SCA3 (Machado-Joseph disease) SCA2	Onset in 20s–30s Nonambulatory within 20 yr after onset Lifespan variably decreased	SCA1: AD/6p SCA3: AD/14q SCA2: AD/12q	Progressive gait ataxia, later involving all limbs; dysarthria, nystagmus, ophthalmoparesis Spasticity, extrapyramidal movement disorders, peripheral neuropathy Variable cognitive impairment
SCA7	Wide age range of onset Childhood onset: death within 5 yr Adult onset: wheelchair-bound within 15 yr	AD/3	Progressive ataxia with visual failure due to macular degeneration Childhood onset: rapidly progressive disease with visual loss, ataxia, seizures, myoclonus, dementia, extrapyramidal symptoms Adult onset: ataxia, brisk reflexes, visual loss, and slow saccades
SCA6 SCA5	Late adult onset (40–50s) Normal lifespan	SCA6: AD/19 SCA5: AD/11p	Pure cerebellar syndrome without involvement of other systems as in other SCA diseases

There are many inherited causes of degenerative ataxia; some of the more important causes are listed here. Note that controversy surrounds the classification of the dominantly inherited ataxias: They are listed here by genotype, although some would include them under the rubric of olivo-ponto-cerebellar atrophy (OPCA). The SCAs are grouped according to similar clinical presentations and are listed in each group in order of decreasing incidence. (Other SCA gene diseases with limited kindreds are not shown here.) Note that all SCAs shown here are dominantly inherited and are due to expanded trinucleotide repeats in the affected gene. Friedreich's ataxia also is a trinucleotide repeat disease but has a unique triplet expansion (GAA) and is recessively inherited.

Evidente et al. (2000); Subramony, Vig, McDaniel (1999).

REFERENCES

Belay ED. Transmissible spongiform encephalopathies in humans. *Annu Rev Microbiol.* 1999;53:283–314.

Bentes C, Carvalho M, Evangelista T, Sales-Luis ML. Multifocal motor neuropathy mimicking motor neuron disease: Nine cases. *J Neurol Sci.* 1999;169:76–79.

Biros I, Forrest S. Spinal muscular atrophy: Untangling the knot? *J Med Genet.* 1999;36:1–8.

Bouche P, Le Forestier N, Maisonobe T, Fournier E, Wiler JC. Electrophysiological diagnosis of motor neuron disease and pure motor neuropathy. *J Neurol.* 1999;246:520–525.

Brooks BR. Clinical epidemiology of amyotrophic lateral sclerosis. *Neurol Clin.* 1996;14:400–420.

Brooks BR. Defining optimal management in ALS: From first symptoms to announcement. *Neurology.* 1999;53:S1–S3.

Chaudhry V. Multifocal motor neuropathy. *Semin Neurol.* 1998;18:73–81.

Cole N, Siddique T. Genetic disorders of motor neurons. *Semin Neurol.* 1999;19:407–418.

Dimauro S, Bonilla E. Mitochondrial encephalomyopathies. In: Rosenberg RN, Prusiner SB, eds. *The Molecular and Genetic Basis of Neurological Diseases.* Boston: Butterworth-Heinemann; 1997:201–235.

DiMauro S, Schon EA. Mitochondrial DNA and diseases of the nervous system: The spectrum. *The Neuroscientist.* 1998;4:53–63.

Evidente VG, Gwinn-Hardy KA, Caviness JN, Gilman S. Hereditary ataxias. *Mayo Clin Proc.* 2000;75:475–490.

Geyer JD, Keating JM, Potts DC. *Neurology for the Boards.* Philadelphia: Lippincott-Raven; 1998:231–268.

Jackson CE, Bryan WW. Amyotrophic lateral sclerosis. *Semin Neurol.* 1998;18:27–39.

Liang BC. Alzheimer's disease. In: Liang B, Higgins DS, Paskavitz J, eds. *Hospital Physician: Neurology Board Review Manual.* Wayne, PA: Turner White Communications; 1998:1–56.

McArthur JC, Sacktor N, Selnes O. Human immunodeficiency virus-associated dementia. *Semin Neurol.* 1999;19:129–150.

Perkin GD. Parkinsonian syndromes. In: Perkin GD, ed. *An Atlas of Parkinson's disease and Related Disorders.* New York: Parthenon Publishing Group; 1997:13–34.

Rodnitzky RL. The parkinsonisms: Identifying what is not Parkinson's disease. *The Neurologist.* 1999;5:300–312.

Ross MA. Acquired neuromuscular diseases: Acquired motor neuron disorders. *Neurol Clin.* 1997;15:482–500.

Rowland LP. Diagnosis of amyotrophic lateral sclerosis. *J Neurol Sci.* 1998; 160:S6–S24.

So YT, Simon RP. Deficiency diseases of the nervous system. In: Bradley WG, Daroff RB, Fenichel GM, Marsden CD, eds. *Neurology in Clinical Practice*. 3rd ed. Boston: Butterworth-Heinemann; 2000:1495–1510.

Subramony SH, Vig PJS, McDaniel DO. Dominantly inherited ataxias. *Semin Neurol*. 1999;19:419–425.

8

Muscle and Neuromuscular Junction Disorders

Kanokwan Boonyapisit and Henry J. Kaminski

Categories of Muscle Disease

Category	Acute or Subacute Weakness	Chronic Generalized Weakness
Hereditary	Metabolic and mitochondrial myopathies	Duchenne's or Becker's, limb-girdle, facioscapulohumeral, myotonic, and other dystrophies, metabolic and mitochondrial myopathies
Inflammatory	Polymyositis	Polymyositis and other inflammatory myopathies, including sarcoidosis
Infectious	Viral (echo, influenza, HIV), parasite (trichinosis)	Viral (HIV), parasite (toxoplasmosis)
Endocrine	Hypocalcemic tetany	Hypo- and hyperthyroidism, hyperparathyroidism, Cushing's and Addison's disease, acromegaly
Toxic	Critical illness, drugs	Alcohol, corticosteroids, zidovudine, etc.
Nutritional		Cachectic myopathy
Channelopathies	Hyper- and hypokalemic periodic paralyses, myotonias	
Neuromuscular junction	Myasthenia gravis, botulism, magnesium toxicity, drugs, rarely Lambert-Eaton myasthenic syndrome	Myasthenia gravis, Lambert-Eaton myasthenic syndrome, congenital myasthenic syndromes

Griggs, Mendell, and Miller (1995).

Muscular Dystrophy

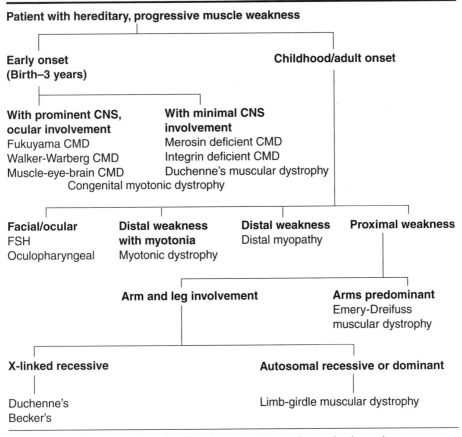

CMD: congenital muscular dystrophy; FSH: facioscapulohumeral muscular dystrophy.

Kissel and Mendell (1999); Tsao and Mendell (1999).

Muscular Dystrophies Caused by Disorders of Sarcolemmal Proteins

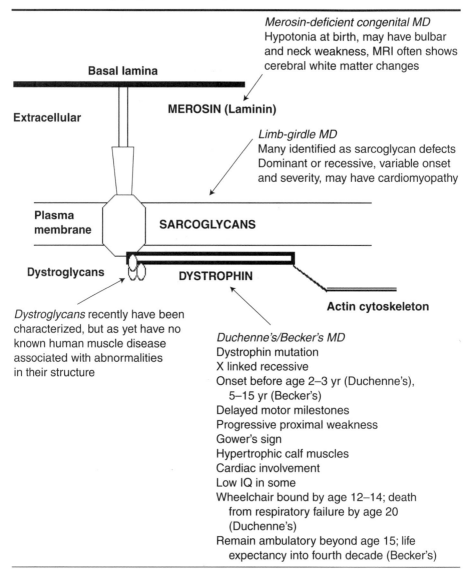

Basal lamina

Merosin-deficient congenital MD
Hypotonia at birth, may have bulbar
and neck weakness, MRI often shows
cerebral white matter changes

Extracellular

MEROSIN (Laminin)

Limb-girdle MD
Many identified as sarcoglycan defects
Dominant or recessive, variable onset
and severity, may have cardiomyopathy

**Plasma
membrane**

SARCOGLYCANS

Dystroglycans

DYSTROPHIN

Actin cytoskeleton

Dystroglycans recently have been
characterized, but as yet have no
known human muscle disease
associated with abnormalities
in their structure

Duchenne's/Becker's MD
Dystrophin mutation
X linked recessive
Onset before age 2–3 yr (Duchenne's),
　　5–15 yr (Becker's)
Delayed motor milestones
Progressive proximal weakness
Gower's sign
Hypertrophic calf muscles
Cardiac involvement
Low IQ in some
Wheelchair bound by age 12–14; death
　　from respiratory failure by age 20
　　(Duchenne's)
Remain ambulatory beyond age 15; life
　　expectancy into fourth decade (Becker's)

Molnar and Karpati (1999).

Toxic Causes of Myopathy

Agent	Clinical Presentation
Alcohol	Three forms: Rhabdomyolysis (occurs in setting of muscle injury related to seizures, coma, hypokalemia, or hypophosphatemia) Acute painful myopathy Chronic alcoholic myopathy (often associated with neuropathy, may be nutritional in origin)
Cocaine	Acute rhabdomyolysis associated with severe muscle pain
Corticosteroid	Subacute, chronic proximal myopathy usually associated with signs of steroid excess (weight gain, moon facies, etc.) Severe acute myopathy is associated with high-dose IV steroid treatment in the intensive care setting.
Thyroid hormone	Proximal myopathy; surreptitious or excess replacement of thyroid hormone should be considered in the appropriate clinical setting
Colchicine	Proximal, painless myopathy with marked elevation of creatine kinase (CK), may occur with overdose or in the presence of renal failure
Cyclosporine	Associated with myalgia and mild elevations of CK; myotonia may occur; occurs more commonly in association with use of cholesterol lowering agents
Lovastatin, clofibrate, and other cholesterol-lowering agents	Acute or subacute, painful myopathy with elevated CK More common among patients with renal failure
Zidovudine	Proximal, painless myopathy related to mitochondrial toxicity Ragged red fibers may be identified with vacuolization
Intramuscular injections	Any IM injection may lead to serum CK elevation; repeated injections lead to local induration and fibrosis Meperidine and pentazocine injection often is associated with abscess formation

Argov and Mastaglia (1994).

Adult Idiopathic Inflammatory Myopathy

Disease	Clinical Presentation	Systemic Manifestation	Laboratory Investigations	Treatment
Adult dermato-myositis	Proximal weakness, myalgia Dysphagia Weakness of neck flexion Heliotropic, erythematous rash around the eyes	Cardiac arrhythmia, peri-carditis, myocarditis, interstitial lung disease, vasculitis of the GI tract Associated with malig-nancy	Elevated CK Positive ANA in 24–60% Positive anti-Jo-1 (associated with lung disease) EMG: increased insertional activity, myopathic motor unit action poten-tials Muscle biopsy: perifascicular atrophy, inflammatory cells in perivascular and perimysium	Corticosteroids, azathioprine, methotrexate, cyclosporine, IVIG Evaluation for possible malignancy
Polymyositis	Proximal weakness, dys-phagia, weakness of neck flexion No skin lesions	Cardiac arrhythmia, peri-carditis, myocarditis, interstitial lung disease, polyarthritis Association with malig-nancy less than in der-matomyositis	Similar to dermatomyositis Muscle biopsy: necrotic and regenerat-ing fibers, endomesial inflammation with invasion of the nonnecrotic fibers	Same as for dermato-myositis
Inclusion body myositis	Slowly progressive proximal and distal weakness Usually involves quadriceps and volar forearm muscles (wrist and finger flexors) Muscle wasting Dysphagia may occur Onset in late adulthood Men affected more often than women	No involvement of other systems No association with malignancy	Normal or mildly elevated CK EMG: increased insertional activity, small, short-duration (myopathic) motor units or large polyphasic motor units Muscle biopsy: endomysial inflamma-tion, muscle fibers with rimmed vac-uole lined with granular material EM: cytoplasmic or intranuclear tubulofilaments	Does not respond well to immune modulat-ing therapy Minimal response to IVIG

Inclusion body myositis often is confused with polymyositis, but weakness of finger and wrist flexors is a hallmark, in addition to its poor response to corticosteroids. The association of dermatomyositis with malignancy is well established but that with polymyositis is less so.

Amato and Barohn (1997).

Metabolic Myopathy

Disease	Clinical Presentation	Laboratory Investigations
Disorders of glycogen		
Acid maltase deficiency	Infancy–adulthood Presentations range from severe, progressive neuropathy in infants to mild myopathy in adults (adults may present with isolated respiratory failure), hypotonia, cardiomegaly, hepatomegaly, enlarged tongue (much less prominent in adults) Autosomal recessive	Elevated CK EMG: myotonic, complex repetitive discharges Muscle biopsy: vacuolar myopathy with glycogen storage Glycogen deposition in skeletal muscles, heart, liver, brain cells, motor neurons (deposition is most prominent in adult forms) Acid maltase deficiency in muscles, liver, heart, cultured fibroblasts
Myophosphorylase deficiency (McArdle's disease)	Childhood onset but often not diagnosed until second–third decade Exercise intolerance, often after brief intense exercise, myalgia, stiffness or weakness of exercising muscles and relief by rest Rhabdomyolysis/myoglobinuria after exercise Autosomal recessive, rarely dominant	Elevated CK; attacks of myoglobinuria have markedly elevated CK EMG: normal between attacks Ischemic exercise test: no elevation of lactate Muscle biopsy: subsarcolemmal deposition of glycogen Negative histochemical stain for myophosphorylase
Disorders of lipids		
Carnitine palmitoyl transferase deficiency (CPT deficiency)	Childhood or young adult Myalgia, muscle stiffness triggered by prolonged exercise, infection, cold, stress, low-carbohydrate/high-fat diet Muscle strength usually normal between the attacks Autosomal recessive, male predominance	Normal CK between attacks, but elevated during attacks and when myoglobinuria occurs Ischemic exercise test: normal EMG: normal (between attacks) Muscle biopsy: decreased CPT activity, otherwise normal
Carnitine deficiency	Childhood/young adult Progressive muscle weakness Cardiomyopathy, hypoglycemia Autosomal recessive	Elevated CK Ischemic exercise test: normal EMG: myopathic changes Muscle biopsy: increased lipid storage, decreased carnitine Decreased carnitine in blood, muscles, liver, kidney

Metabolic myopathies often are suggested by muscle pain and weakness after exercise. Some major causes are shown here.

Dimauro and Bruno (1998); Dimauro and Tsujino (1994); Ziers (1994).

Mitochondrial Diseases with Prominent Muscle Weakness

Syndrome	Clinical Features	Genetics
Chronic progressive external ophthalmoplegia (CPEO)	Ptosis, limited eye movement, mild proximal myopathy, Kearns-Sayre syndrome (pigmented retinopathy, heart block, and external ophthalmoplegia), ragged red fibers on trichrome stain	Maternal inheritance with mitochondrial DNA (mtDNA) deletion Some forms are autosomal dominant
Mitochondrial encephalomyopathy with lactic acidosis, and strokelike episodes (MELAS)	Proximal myopathy with ragged red fibers Acute recurrent focal neurological deficits Progressive encephalopathy Focal or generalized seizures, dementia, headache	Point mutation of tRNA gene in mitochondrial genome
Myoclonus epilepsy with ragged red fibers (MERRF)	Proximal myopathy with ragged red fibers, myoclonus, cerebellar ataxia, seizures, deafness, vascular headache, peripheral neuropathy	Point mutation of tRNA gene in mitochondrial genome
Myo-neuro-gastrointestinal encephalopathy (MNGIE)	Myopathy, peripheral neuropathy, gastrointestinal pseudo-obstruction	Multiple mtDNA mutations
Neurogenic weakness, ataxia, retinitis pigmentosa (NARP)	Sensory neuropathy, ataxia, dementia, retinitis pigmentosa Weakness and atrophy not related to muscle involvement	mtDNA protein coding gene mutation

Mitochondrial disorders have remarkably varied presentations. They should be considered when there is evidence of multiorgan system involvement. The combination of ophthalmoparesis and muscle weakness suggests a mitochondrial myopathy (as long as a neuromuscular transmission disorder is not present).

Morgan-Hughes (1994); Dimauro and Bonilla (1997).

Channelopathies and Myotonias

Disease	Clinical Features	Provocative Factors	Mutation	Treatment
Hypokalemic periodic paralysis	Attacks of general weakness	Heavy exercise Carbohydrate load	L-type calcium channel	K⁺ replacement Avoid provocatives
Thyrotoxic hypokalemic periodic paralysis	Attacks of general weakness	Thyrotoxicosis	Unknown	K⁺ replacement Treat thyroid disorder
Hyperkalemic periodic paralysis	Attacks of general weakness (brief)	Rest after exercise Cold, general anesthesia, sleep	Skeletal muscle sodium channel	Acetazolamide Frequent high-carbohydrate meals
Paramyotonia congenita	Attacks of general weakness, myotonia, muscle stiffness	Cold Prolonged exercise	Skeletal muscle sodium channel	Keep muscles warm Mexiletine
Myotonia congenita*	Myotonia Usually normal strength Muscle hypertrophy	Myotonia provoked by activity but decreases with continued activity	Skeletal muscle chloride channel	Rarely needs treatment but can use mexiletine, phenytoin
Myotonic dystrophy	Progressive myopathy with facial weakness, myotonia, diabetes, cataracts, other systemic signs	Percussion and grip myotonia	Trinucleotide repeat of myotonin, a protein kinase	Supportive for complications of weakness and systemic manifestations
Proximal myotonic myopathy	Progressive myopathy, myotonia, cataracts	Mild percussion and grip myotonia	Unknown	Supportive; myotonia may require treatment

*Clinical variants: Thomsen's disease presents in childhood and is milder; Becker myotonia more often leads to a progressive myopathy.

The periodic paralyses may be easily differentiated by the differences in the length of attacks and their provocative factors.

Barchi (1997, 1998).

Neuromuscular Transmission Disorders

Disorder	Clinical Presentation	Pathogenesis	Diagnosis	Treatment	Comments
Myasthenia gravis	Fluctuating signs of ptosis, diplopia, dysarthria, dysphagia, limb weakness, respiratory insufficiency	Antibodies against the skeletal muscle acetylcholine receptor (AChR)	80–90% have decremental response with slow stimulation AChR antibodies in 80–90% of generalized and 50% of ocular patients. Tensilon test (false positives seen in brainstem tumors, ALS, and other neuromuscular transmission disorders)	Pyridostigmine, immunosuppression, plasma exchange or IVIG for severe weakness, thymectomy (10% have thymoma)	Remarkably varied presentations; perform fatiguing maneuvers to bring out weakness on exam
Lambert-Eaton myasthenic syndrome	Proximal (variable ocular and bulbar) weakness, dry mouth, orthostasis, reduced pupillary light reflex	Antibodies to calcium channels and possibly other proteins	Decreased compound muscle action potential (CMAP) amplitude, incremental response to rapid stimulation, P/Q channel antibodies found in nearly all patients with cancer and most non-paraneoplastic patients	3,4-diaminopyridine, pyridostigmine, immunosuppression. Treatment of associated malignancy may improve neurologic complaints	At least 60% of patients have cancer, usually small cell lung cancer
Botulism	Descending bulbar paralysis with autonomic dysfunction	Toxin produced by *Clostridium botulinum* cleaves synaptic proteins at motor and autonomic cholinergic nerve terminals	CMAP reduced; variable response to repetitive stimulation; incremental response may not be seen. Culture of *C. botulinum* or detection of toxin	Supportive care; antiserum not of proven benefit	Consider with wound infections, postop patients, and among IV drug abusers

| Congenital myasthenic syndromes | Ranges from profound weakness at birth to presentation in adulthood | AChR subunit, acetylcholinesterase, and likely other gene mutations | Decremental response with slow repetitive stimulation Confirmation requires extensive molecular and physiologic testing | Supportive care; pyridostigmine and quinidine sulfate help in some patients | Rare, but think of this in the seronegative patient with a long history and signs of fatigue |

Middleton (1999); Boonyapisit, Kaminski, and Ruff (1999).

Medications That Worsen (or Unmask) Myasthenia Gravis

Medication	Comment
Prednisone	A common treatment for MG, but started at high doses will make about half of patients worse.
Aminoglycosides and other antibiotics	The aminoglycosides frequently will weaken the myasthenic. Reports exist of nearly every antibiotic worsening myasthenia, but the majority of patients never have problems.
Quinidine, procainamide	Several cardiovascular drugs are reported to worsen myasthenia, these two most consistently. Quinine, still found in some tonic waters, also worsens myasthenia.
Magnesium	Magnesium inhibits calcium-mediated release of acetylcholine. The most common sources of magnesium are antacid preparations.
D-penicillamine	Induces an autoimmune response, most commonly seen in patients treated for rheumatoid arthritis. With discontinuation of treatment, myasthenia usually resolves.
Other	Lithium, phenytoin, inhalation anesthetics, contrast agents for radiographic imaging.

Howard (1990).

Intensive Care Patient with Weakness

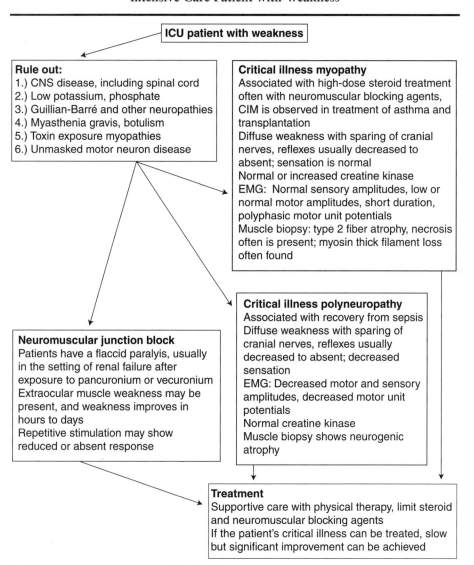

ICU patient with weakness

Rule out:
1.) CNS disease, including spinal cord
2.) Low potassium, phosphate
3.) Guillian-Barré and other neuropathies
4.) Myasthenia gravis, botulism
5.) Toxin exposure myopathies
6.) Unmasked motor neuron disease

Critical illness myopathy
Associated with high-dose steroid treatment often with neuromuscular blocking agents, CIM is observed in treatment of asthma and transplantation
Diffuse weakness with sparing of cranial nerves, reflexes usually decreased to absent; sensation is normal
Normal or increased creatine kinase
EMG: Normal sensory amplitudes, low or normal motor amplitudes, short duration, polyphasic motor unit potentials
Muscle biopsy: type 2 fiber atrophy, necrosis often is present; myosin thick filament loss often found

Critical illness polyneuropathy
Associated with recovery from sepsis
Diffuse weakness with sparing of cranial nerves, reflexes usually decreased to absent; decreased sensation
EMG: Decreased motor and sensory amplitudes, decreased motor unit potentials
Normal creatine kinase
Muscle biopsy shows neurogenic atrophy

Neuromuscular junction block
Patients have a flaccid paralyis, usually in the setting of renal failure after exposure to pancuronium or vecuronium
Extraocular muscle weakness may be present, and weakness improves in hours to days
Repetitive stimulation may show reduced or absent response

Treatment
Supportive care with physical therapy, limit steroid and neuromuscular blocking agents
If the patient's critical illness can be treated, slow but significant improvement can be achieved

Lacoumis (1998).

Hypotonic Infant

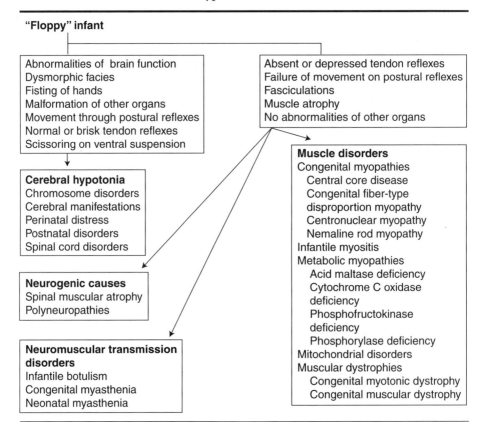

"Floppy" infant

| Abnormalities of brain function
Dysmorphic facies
Fisting of hands
Malformation of other organs
Movement through postural reflexes
Normal or brisk tendon reflexes
Scissoring on ventral suspension | Absent or depressed tendon reflexes
Failure of movement on postural reflexes
Fasciculations
Muscle atrophy
No abnormalities of other organs |

Cerebral hypotonia
Chromosome disorders
Cerebral manifestations
Perinatal distress
Postnatal disorders
Spinal cord disorders

Neurogenic causes
Spinal muscular atrophy
Polyneuropathies

Neuromuscular transmission disorders
Infantile botulism
Congenital myasthenia
Neonatal myasthenia

Muscle disorders
Congenital myopathies
  Central core disease
  Congenital fiber-type
  disproportion myopathy
  Centronuclear myopathy
  Nemaline rod myopathy
Infantile myositis
Metabolic myopathies
  Acid maltase deficiency
  Cytochrome C oxidase
  deficiency
  Phosphofructokinase
  deficiency
  Phosphorylase deficiency
Mitochondrial disorders
Muscular dystrophies
  Congenital myotonic dystrophy
  Congenital muscular dystrophy

Fenichel (1997).

Elevated Creatine Kinase Levels

Sustained asymptomatic CK elevation
   African-American men
   Individuals with large lean muscle mass
   Regular, prolonged, weight-bearing exercise

Transient CK elevation in the absence of neuromuscular disease
   Exercise (prolonged, weight bearing, or among untrained subjects)
   Muscle trauma
   Surgical procedures or intramuscular injection
   Convulsive seizures

Reversible CK elevations
   Metabolic
      Hypothyroidism
      Malignancy
      Nutritional
   Drugs and toxins
      Amphetamines, albuterol, carbimazole, clofibrate, cocaine, colchicine, cyclopropan,
         danazol, digoxin, emetine, ethanol, gemfibrozil, furosemide, halothane, heroin,
         HMG CoA inhibitors (statins), imipramine, ketamine, meperidine, penicillamine,
         phencyclidine, vitamin E, zidovudine

Myopathies associated with marked CK elevation (up to 50–100-fold above normal)
   Dystrophinopathies (Duchenne's and Becker's muscular dystrophies)
   Rhabdomyolysis
   Malignant hyperthermia
   Neuroleptic malignant syndrome
   Polymyositis

Myopathies commonly associated with no or minimal CK elevation
   Steroid myopathy
   Hyperthyroid myopathy
   Mitochondrial myopathy
   Channelopathies (with exception of malignant hyperthermia)

Penn (1994).

Myoglobinuria and Rhabdomyolysis

Metabolic defects
   Carnitine palmitoyltransferase deficiency
   Deficiencies of glycolytic enzymes, such as myophosphorylase, phosphofructokinase
   Mitochondrial diseases
   Myoadenylate deaminase deficiency

Sporadic
   Prolonged exercise in excess of training
   Status epilepticus
   Tetanus
   Agitated delirium
   Electric shock, lightning strike
   Heat stroke
   Malignant hyperthermia
   Neuroleptic malignant syndrome
   Infections
   Drugs and toxins, see *Toxic Causes of Myopathy*

Muscle necrosis
   Crush injury
   Coma
   Toxic

Loss of muscle membrane integrity
   Toxic
   Snake toxins, hornet, wasp and bee venom, staphylococcal toxic shock syndrome

Salt and water imbalances
   Hypokalemia
   Hypernatremia
   Water intoxication
   Hypophosphatemia
   Hyperosmolar nonketotic state

Infections
   Viral: influenza, coxsackie, herpes, adenovirus, HIV
   Bacterial: staphylococcal, typhoid, Legionella, Clostridia, E. coli

Primary myopathies
   Dermatomyositis
   Polymyositis

Penn (1994).

Lesion Localization by Nerve Conduction Studies and Needle EMG

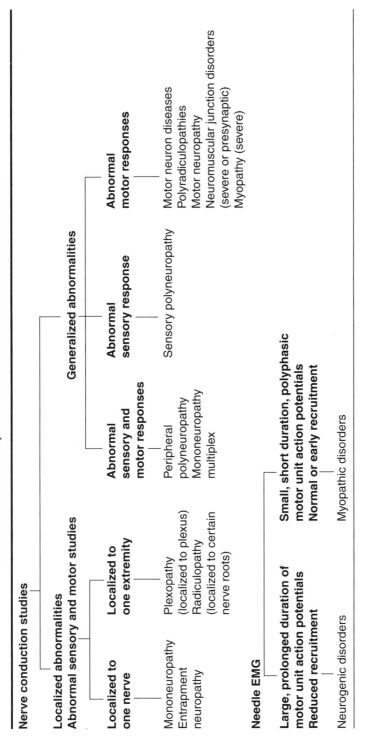

Nerve conduction studies

Localized abnormalities
Abnormal sensory and motor studies

Localized to one nerve	**Localized to one extremity**	**Abnormal sensory and motor responses**	**Abnormal sensory response**	**Abnormal motor responses**
		Generalized abnormalities		
Mononeuropathy	Plexopathy (localized to plexus)	Peripheral polyneuropathy	Sensory polyneuropathy	Motor neuron diseases
Entrapment neuropathy	Radiculopathy (localized to certain nerve roots)	Mononeuropathy multiplex		Polyradiculopathies
				Motor neuropathy
				Neuromuscular junction disorders (severe or presynaptic)
				Myopathy (severe)

Needle EMG

Large, prolonged duration of motor unit action potentials **Reduced recruitment**	**Small, short duration, polyphasic motor unit action potentials** **Normal or early recruitment**
Neurogenic disorders	Myopathic disorders

Note that postsynaptic neuromuscular junction disorders, usually myasthenia gravis, often have normal routine nerve conduction studies and needle EMG examination, but show an abnormal decremental response to slow repetitive stimulation.

Preston and Shapiro (1998).

Pathological Classification of Neuromuscular Disease Based on Nerve Conduction Studies and Needle EMG

	Axonal Disease	Demyelination	Myopathy	Neuromuscular Junction Disorder
Nerve conduction studies				
CMAP amplitude	Reduced	Normal or conduction block	Normal or reduced in severe cases	Normal or reduced in presynaptic disorders
Conduction velocity	Normal or slightly reduced with severe axonal loss	Slow conduction velocity	Normal	Normal
Repetitive stimulation	Normal	Normal	Normal	Decremental response on slow repetitive stimulation in postsynaptic disorders; Incremental response on rapid repetitive stimulation in presynaptic disorders
Needle EMG				
Insertional activity	Increased	Normal	Increased in myopathy with necrosis and destruction of terminal nerve endings, such as inflammatory myopathy; Otherwise normal	Normal
Motor unit action potentials	Large amplitude, prolonged duration, polyphasic motor unit action potentials with reduced recruitment	Normal or minimal changes due to associated secondary axonal loss; Decreased recruitment in the presence of conduction block	Short-duration, small-amplitude, polyphasic motor unit action potentials with normal or early recruitment	Normal

CMAP: compound muscle action potential.

REFERENCES

Amato AA, Barohn RJ. Idiopathic inflammatory myopathies. *Neurol Clin.* 1997;15:615–648.

Argov Z, Mastaglia FL. Drug-induced neuromuscular disorders in man. In: Walton J, Karpati G, Hilton-Jones D, eds. *Disorders of Voluntary Muscle.* Edinburgh: Churchill Livingstone; 1994:989–1032.

Barchi RL. Molecular pathology of the periodic paralyses. In: Rosenberg RN, Prusiner SB, eds. *The Molecular and Genetic Basis of Neurological Diseases.* Boston: Butterworth-Heinemann; 1997:723–731.

Barchi RL. Ion channel mutations affecting muscle and brain. *Curr Opin Neurol.* 1998;11:461–468.

Boonyapisit K, Kaminski HJ, Ruff RL. The molecular basis of neuromuscular transmission disorders. *Am J Med.* 1999;106:97–113.

Dimauro S, Bonilla E. Mitochondrial encephalomyopathies. In: Rosenberg RN, Prusiner SB, eds. *The Molecular and Genetic Basis of Neurological Diseases.* Boston: Butterworth-Heinemann: 1997:201–235.

Dimauro S, Bruno C. Glycogen storage diseases of muscle. *Curr Opin Neurol.* 1998;11:477–484.

Dimauro S, Tsujino S. Nonlysosomal glycogenoses. In: Engel AG, Franzini-Armstrong C, eds. *Myology.* New York: McGraw-Hill; 1994:1554–1575.

Fenichel GM. *Clinical Pediatric Neurology.* Philadelphia: W.B. Saunders Co.; 1997:176–204.

Griggs RC, Mendell JR, Miller RG. *Evaluation and Treatment of Myopathies.* Philadelphia: F.A. Davis; 1995:17–78.

Howard JF. Adverse drug effects on neuromuscular transmission. *Semin Neurol.* 1990;10:89–102.

Kissel JT, Mendell JR. Muscular dystrophy: Historical overview and classification in the genetic era. *Semin Neurol.* 1999;19:5–7.

Middleton LT. Disorders of the neuromuscular junction. In: Schapira AHV, Griggs RC, eds. *Muscle Diseases.* Boston: Butterworth-Heinemann; 1999:251–297.

Molnar MJ, Karpati G. Muscular dystrophies related to deficiency of sarcolemmal proteins. In: Schapira AHV, Griggs RC, eds. *Muscle Diseases.* Boston: Butterworth-Heinemann; 1999:83–114.

Morgan-Hughes JA. Mitochondrial diseases. In: Engel AG, Franzini-Armstrong C, eds. *Myology.* New York: McGraw-Hill; 1994:1610–1660.

Penn AS. Myoglobinuria. In: Engel AG, Franzini-Armstrong C, eds. *Myology.* New York: McGraw-Hill; 1994:1679–1696.

Preston DC, Shapiro BE. *Electromyography and Neuromuscular Disorders: Clinical-Electrophysiologic Correlation.* Boston: Butterworth-Heinemann; 1998:23–74;143–206.

Tsao CY, Mendell JR. The childhood muscular dystrophies: Making order out of chaos. *Semin Neurol.* 1999;19:9–23.

Ziers S. Carnitine palmitoyltransferase deficiency. In: Engel AG, Franzini-Armstrong C, eds. *Myology.* New York: McGraw-Hill; 1994:1577–1586.

9

Peripheral Neuropathy

Nicholas P. Poolos

Signs and Symptoms of Peripheral Neuropathy

Sign or Symptom	Pattern	Pathology and Examples
Weakness	Symmetric weakness beginning distally in feet, progressing proximally to legs, eventually involving upper extremities. Sensory loss present. Progression over weeks to months.	Sensorimotor neuropathy, usually of axonal pathology, due to metabolic disease, toxins, or vitamin deficiency.
	Rapidly progressive weakness over days involving all extremities, bulbar, and/or cranial muscles. Weakness predominates over sensory loss.	Demyelinating neuropathy, such as Guillain-Barré syndrome, diphtheric neuropathy; CIDP if progression over weeks.
	Acute weakness in muscles supplied by one or several nerves. Sensation may be spared but pain is prominent.	Mononeuropathy multiplex due to vasculitic cause. Diabetes may produce single or multiple entrapment neuropathies.
Sensory loss	Symmetric loss of all sensory modalities beginning in feet and gradually progressing proximally, producing "glove and stocking" deficits. Loss of sensation precedes motor weakness, if any.	Most sensorimotor and sensory neuropathies follow this pattern. Subacute sensory neuropathy is often of idiopathic cause.
Pain	Paresthesias or burning sensations, symmetric with a distal predominance, usually in absence of weakness or significant impairment of other sensory modalities.	Small-fiber axonal pathology, as seen in diabetes or EtOH-induced neuropathy.
Ataxia	Loss of position sense, usually worse in lower extremities. Other sensory modalities spared.	Large-fiber sensory neuropathy, as in Miller Fisher variant of GBS; sensory neuronopathy due to paraneoplastic causes.
Loss of reflexes	Any of the above patterns.	Hallmark of peripheral neuropathy of any cause, with possible exception of small-fiber neuropathies in early stages.

CIDP: chronic inflammatory demyelinating polyneuropathy; GBS: Guillain-Barré syndrome.

Peripheral neuropathy usually is marked by symmetric weakness and sensory loss that begins in the distal lower extremities and gradually progresses proximally. After affecting the lower extremities up to the knee, sensory symptoms begin to appear in the hands. With further progression, the trunk may begin to be affected, starting in the midline. Notable exceptions to this pattern are the rapidly ascending diffuse pathology of the inflammatory polyradiculopathies, such as Guillain-Barré syndrome, and the asymmetric involvement of mononeuropathy multiplex. See also *Diagnosis of Peripheral Neuropathy* and *Peripheral Neuropathy with Distinctive Patterns.*

Adams, Victor, and Ropper (1997); Barohn (1998).

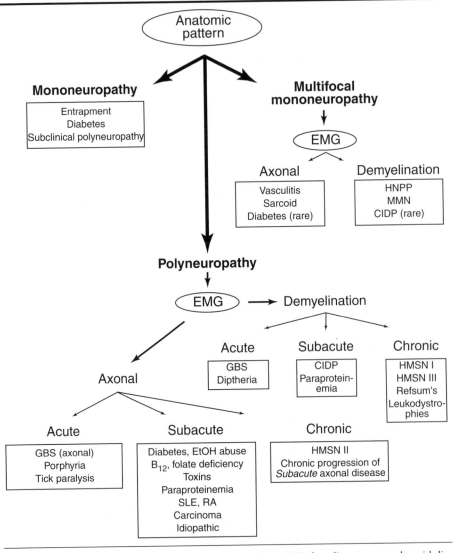

CIDP: chronic inflammatory demyelinating polyneuropathy; HNPP: hereditary neuropathy with liability to pressure palsy; GBS: Guillain-Barré syndrome; HMSN: hereditary motor and sensory neuropathy; MMN: multifocal motor neuropathy.

The diagnosis of peripheral neuropathy can be approached by identifying the anatomic pattern and the time course, then incorporating EMG data. The diseases shown in each category comprise some of the common causes in that category but are not an exhaustive list. See also *Lesion Localization by Nerve Conduction Studies and Needle EMG*, in Chapter 8.

Modified with permission from Asbury AK, Tomas PK. The clinical approach to neuropathy. In: Asbury AK, Thomas PK, eds. *Peripheral Nerve Disorders 2*. Oxford: Butterworth-Heinemann; 1995:1–28.

Peripheral Neuropathy by Clinical Course

Acute onset (within days)	Guillain-Barré syndrome Acute intermittent porphyria Critical illness polyneuropathy Diphtheric neuropathy Thallium toxicity
Subacute onset (weeks to months)	Toxins or medications Nutritional deficiency Metabolic abnormality Paraneoplastic syndrome CIDP
Chronic course (years)	Hereditary motor and sensory neuropathy (HMSN) Dominantly inherited sensory neuropathy CIDP
Relapsing/remitting course	Guillain-Barré syndrome CIDP HIV/AIDS Toxins (intermittent exposure) Porphyria

CIDP: chronic inflammatory demyelinating polyneuropathy.

Modified with permission from Poncelet AN. An algorithm for the evaluation of peripheral neuropathy. *Am Fam Physician.* 1998.

Peripheral Neuropathy with Distinctive Patterns

Predominantly motor weakness	Guillain-Barré syndrome
	CIDP
	Hereditary motor and sensory neuropathy (HMSN)
	Multifocal motor neuropathy with conduction block
	Porphyria
	Toxins: vincristine, dapsone, lead
Purely sensory loss	Miller Fisher syndrome
	Paraneoplastic sensory neuronopathy (anti-Hu)
	Cis-platinum toxicity
	Sjögren's syndrome
	MGUS
With significant pain	Diabetes
	Vasculitis
	Alcohol
	Toxins: arsenic, thallium
	Amyloid
	Paraneoplastic sensory neuronopathy (anti-Hu)
	HIV-related distal symmetric polyneuropathy
	Idiopathic distal small-fiber neuropathy
Involving upper limbs predominantly	Guillain-Barré syndrome
	Diabetes
	Porphyria
	B_{12} deficiency
	Lead toxicity
Involving cranial nerves	Diabetes
	Guillain-Barré syndrome
	HIV/AIDS
	Lyme disease
	Sarcoidosis
	Meningeal carcinomatosis
	Diphtheria

CIDP: Chronic inflammatory demyelinating polyradiculoneuropathy; MGUS: Monoclonal gammopathy of undetermined significance.

Bosch and Mitsumoto (1996); Thomas and Ochoa (1993).

Axonal vs. Demyelinating Neuropathy

	Axonal Degeneration	*Segmental Demyelination*
Motor nerve conduction studies		
CMAP amplitude	Decreased	Normal (except with conduction block)
Distal latency	Normal	Prolonged
Conduction velocity	Normal	Slow
Conduction block	Absent	Present
Temporal dispersion	Absent	Present
F wave	Normal	Prolonged or absent
H reflex	Normal	Prolonged or absent
Sensory nerve conduction studies		
SNAP amplitude	Decreased	Normal
Distal latency	Normal	Prolonged
Conduction velocity	Normal	Slow
Needle EMG		
Fibrillations/fasciculations	Present	Absent
Motor unit recruitment	Decreased	Decreased
Motor unit morphology	Long duration, polyphasic	Normal

CMAP: compound muscle action potential; SNAP: sensory nerve action potential.

The pathological basis underlying peripheral neuropathy can be divided into axonal and demyelinating causes. Both can cause weakness and sensory loss in the distribution of the affected nerve, the former through loss of axons in the nerve, the latter through blockade of action potential conduction at sites of segmental demyelination. These categories of pathology can be distinguished by their differing electrophysiological characteristics.

Modified with permission from Barohn RJ. Approach to peripheral neuropathy and neuronopathy. *Semin Neurol.* 1998;18:12.

Neuropathy Associated with Paraproteinemia

Paraprotein	Disease	EMG Features	Systemic Features
IgG-κ or IgM-κ or IgA-κ <3 g/dl	Monoclonal gammopathy of undetermined significance (MGUS)	Demyelinating or axonal	Distinguished from MM by absence of systemic features and Ig <3 g/dl 20% progress to plasma cell dyscrasia
IgM-κ or IgG-κ >3 g/dl	Multiple myeloma (MM)	Axonal	Bone pain, fatigue, anemia, hypercalcemia, renal insufficiency
IgM-κ	Waldenstrom's macroglobulinemia	Demyelinating	Fatigue, weight loss, oronasal bleeding, blurred vision, encephalopathy
IgM or IgG	Lymphoma	Demyelinating or axonal	Fatigue, weight loss, lymphadenopathy, POEMS syndrome
IgM or IgG	Cryoglobulinemia	Axonal	Hepatosplenomegaly, purpura, arthralgias, leg ulcers, Raynaud's phenomenon
IgG-λ or IgA-λ	Osteosclerotic myeloma	Demyelinating	POEMS syndrome, Castleman's disease
IgG-λ or IgA-λ	Amyloidosis	Axonal	Congestive heart failure, renal failure, hepatosplenomegaly, macroglossia, weight loss

POEMS: polyneuropathy, organomegaly, endocrinopathy, M-protein, and skin changes.

Paraproteins are elevated levels of serum immunoglobulins, usually representing a monoclonal expansion of plasma cells, which have been associated with neuropathy and a variety of systemic disorders. Approximately 10% of peripheral neuropathy is due to paraproteinemia, which can be detected by serum immunoelectrophoresis. Of the paraproteinemias, two-thirds consists of monoclonal gammopathy of undetermined significance (MGUS), in which neuropathy is not associated with a systemic disorder; of this group, approximately 20% subsequently will progress to a plasma cell malignancy (usually multiple myeloma).

Modified with permission from Ropper AH, Gorson KC. Neuropathies associated with paraproteinemia. *New Engl J Med.* 1998.

Toxic Causes of Peripheral Neuropathy

Cause	Clinical Features
Alcohol	Most common cause of nutritional polyneuropathy. Unclear which vitamin deficiency (thiamine, pyridoxine, folate, etc.) is the primary cause.
Arsenic	Associated with gastrointestinal complaints, jaundice, and white banding of the nails (Mee's lines).
Lead	Usually found with chronic industrial exposure, producing distal upper extremity motor weakness (most typically, wrist drop from radial nerve involvement).
Thallium	Toxicity results from accidental exposure to rodenticide, usually in children. Neuropathy is a painful, predominantly sensory polyneuropathy.
Isoniazid (INH)	Polyneuropathy was a common occurrence with INH treatment of tuberculosis, due to its blockade of pyridoxine metabolism. Coadministration with pyridoxine prevents this disorder.
Vincristine	Causes a distal polyneuropathy with motor predominance.
Cis-platinum, paclitaxel	Predominantly sensory polyneuropathy that may begin several weeks after cessation of therapy.
Dapsone	Predominantly motor neuropathy seen with chronic administration for leprosy.
Phenytoin	Treatment with phenytoin over many years can lead to a mild, predominantly sensory, distal neuropathy.

A symmetrical polyneuropathy that evolves in a subacute fashion, over weeks to several months, and then persists most often is due to a toxic or metabolic cause. The underlying pathology usually shows axonal features. Although neuropathy associated with paraneoplastic causes tends to develop over somewhat longer periods of time, it can present within weeks (particularly true of lymphoma) and always should be ruled out.

Adams, Victor, and Ropper (1997).

Autonomic Neuropathy

Disease	Clinical Features
Diabetes mellitus (DM)	Autonomic involvement is common in DM, manifested by postural hypotension, poor heart rate control, impotence, and impaired sweating. The resulting vasomotor and cardiac dysfunction significantly reduces long-term survival.
Amyloidosis	Autonomic dysfunction may precede the motor/sensory loss in this disease and can become disabling.
Guillain-Barré syndrome	Dysautonomia can lead to wide swings in blood pressure and heart rate, particularly in the severely affected patient who is intubated due to respiratory compromise. Cardiac tachyarrhythmia can lead to sudden death.
Porphyria	Hypertension and persistent tachycardia may be the earliest manifestations of neuropathy, owing to dysfunction of the parasympathetic autonomic fibers.
Familial dysautonomia (Riley-Day syndrome)	An autosomal recessively inherited disease manifested by postural hypotension, decreased tearing, hyperhidrosis, poor temperature control, and intermittent skin blotching.

Nerves mediating autonomic function are compromised to some extent by many of the diseases causing peripheral neuropathy but are significantly affected in the diseases shown here. Symptoms of autonomic neuropathy include orthostatic hypotension, dysregulation of heart rate, hyperhidrosis, bladder dysfunction, and impotence in men. Because autonomic fibers are not routinely accessible to neurophysiological testing, demonstration of autonomic neuropathy is limited to testing of autonomic function. This may be done by recording orthostatic blood pressure measurements, sweat testing, and measuring plasma norepinephrine levels.

McLeod (1992).

Multifocal Motor Neuropathy

Clinical Features	MMN	CIDP	ALS
LMN weakness	Distal, asymmetrical	Proximal and distal	Progressive
UMN signs	Absent	Absent	Present
Sensory loss	Absent	Present	Absent
Motor conduction block	Always	Frequent	Rare and transient
Sensory conduction	Normal	Low to absent	Normal
CSF protein	Normal	Elevated	Normal
Anti-GM$_1$ antibodies	80%	Absent	<15%

LMN: lower motor neuron; UMN: upper motor neuron.

The causes of progressive limb weakness with atrophy and no sensory symptoms form a list mainly limited to multifocal motor neuropathy (MMN) with conduction block, chronic inflammatory demyelinating polyradiculoneuropathy (CIDP), and amyotrophic lateral sclerosis (ALS). Although ALS should be distinguishable from the others on the basis of upper motor neuron signs, its grave prognosis requires careful exclusion of these other, more treatable diseases. Other acquired causes of multifocal motor neuropathy include lead or dapsone toxicity, and postpolio syndrome. See also *Diagnosis of Amyotrophic Lateral Sclerosis*, in Chapter 7.

Reprinted with permission Bosch EP, Mitsumoto H. Disorders of peripheral nerves. In: Bradley WG, Daroff RB, Fenichel GM, Marsden CD, eds. *Neurology in Clinical Practice*. 2nd ed. Boston: Butterworth-Heinemann; 1996:1920.

Inherited Causes of Sensorimotor Neuropathy

Disease	Clinical Features
Hereditary motor and sensory neuropathy type I (HMSN type I; CMT type I)	Slow progression of distal leg weakness with atrophy and sensory loss, usually with onset in teens. Lower extremities show high arched feet and hammertoes. Upper extremities are affected later. Nerve conduction studies show demyelination. Inheritance is autosomal dominant, with three different alleles causing clinically similar disease (Chrs. 1, 17, 22).
Hereditary motor and sensory neuropathy type II (HMSN type II; CMT type II)	Similar to type I except much slower progression, so that it may not have clinical onset until middle age. Nerve pathology has axonal features as opposed to the demyelination associated with type I. Autosomal dominant inheritance associated with Chrs. 1 and 3.
Hereditary motor and sensory neuropathy type III (HMSN type III; CMT type III; Dejerine-Sottas disease)	Severe demyelinating neuropathy of infancy or early childhood, causing weakness and wasting of lower extremities along with polymodal sensory loss. Peripheral nerves are markedly hypertrophic. Inheritance usually is autosomal recessive.
Hereditary neuropathy with liability to pressure palsy (HNPP)	Repeated mononeuropathies at common entrapment sites: common peroneal, ulnar, radial, and median nerves, and the brachial plexus. Usually, there is a coexistent mild symmetrical polyneuropathy. Nerve conduction studies show focal demyelination. Inheritance is autosomal dominant, involving deletion of the PMP-22 gene on chromosome 17, the same gene implicated in the most common subtype of HMSN I.
Familial amyloid polyneuropathy	A diverse set of syndromes characterized by autosomal dominant inheritance of peripheral neuropathy and involvement of other organs by amyloid deposition. Symptoms usually begin insidiously in third decade with distal sensory loss and autonomic involvement. Diagnosis is made by detection of amyloid on sural nerve biopsy.

CMT: Charcot-Marie-Tooth disease.

Bosch and Mitsumoto (1996).

Peripheral Neuropathy in Patients with HIV Infection

Neuropathy Type	Clinical Features
Distal symmetrical polyneuropathy	Burning pain and paresthesias in the feet, associated with mild distal sensory loss. May be detected in up to one-third of patients with AIDS. Vitamin B_{12} deficiency or a history of exposure to drugs causing peripheral neuropathy (isoniazid, vincristine, ddI, or ddC) is common. This is the most common form of peripheral neuropathy in HIV patients.
Inflammatory demyelinating polyneuropathy	Guillain-Barré syndrome (GBS) and CIDP have similar appearances in patients with HIV as in uninfected patients; however, these neuropathies occur more frequently in the HIV-infected than in the general population and usually in patients who are otherwise free of HIV sequelae (GBS may occur at HIV seroconversion). The most notable difference is that HIV patients usually show a CSF lymphocytic pleocytosis of 20–50 cells, whereas this is uncommon in patients without HIV.
Mononeuropathy multiplex	Involvement of multiple individual nerves that can result from several causes. Early in the course of HIV infection, vasculitis is a common cause; in more immunocompromised patients, CMV should be considered. In patients with multiple cranial neuropathies, infectious and neoplastic causes should be ruled out, such as toxoplasmosis and lymphoma.
CMV polyradiculopathy	Rapidly ascending polyradiculopathy leading to lower extremity pain and paresthesias, paraparesis, and bladder dysfunction without signs of myelopathy. Lumbar puncture shows a polymorphonuclear pleocytosis. Usually occurs late in the course of AIDS infection, in conjunction with CMV infection.

CIDP: chronic inflammatory demyelinating polyneuropathy; CMV: cytomegalovirus.

Simpson and Olney (1992).

Chronic Peripheral Neuropathy in Children

Disease	Clinical Features
Hereditary motor and sensory neuropathy type I (HMSN I; CMT type I)	Gait disorder that begins usually in teens, associated with foot deformities: pes cavus and hammertoes. The gait disorder usually presents with difficulty running, gradually progressing to foot drop.
Hereditary motor and sensory neuropathy type II (HMSN II; CMT type II)	Similar to HMSN I, except with slower progression and less disability. HMSN II is distinguished on EMG by an axonal pattern of pathology.
Hereditary motor and sensory neuropathy type III (HMSN III; CMT type III; Dejerine-Sottas disease)	Symptomatic in infancy, with delayed motor milestones and hypotonia. Diffuse weakness with severe sensory loss usually occurs by second decade. Autosomal recessive inheritance.
Hereditary motor and sensory neuropathy type IV (HMSN IV; Refsum disease)	Polyneuropathy associated with retinitis pigmentosa and cerebellar ataxia. Clinical course is variable, with onset from first to third decades. Autosomal recessively inherited disorder of phytanic acid metabolism.
Metachromatic leukodystrophy	Disorder causing central and peripheral nervous system demyelination of varying clinical onset, most frequently in first 2 years of age, causing progressive distal weakness and sensory loss as well as loss of cognitive milestones. Autosomal recessively inherited defect in arylsulfatase A.
Giant axonal neuropathy	Rare autosomal recessive disease causing both central and peripheral demyelination. Usually presents in early childhood with distal muscle atrophy, and progressive cognitive impairment, optic atrophy, and cranial neuropathy.

CMT: Charcot-Marie-Tooth disease.

There are few acquired causes of peripheral neuropathy in children, the most common being Guillain-Barré disease. Chronic peripheral neuropathy in children predominantly is inherited. Note that motor neuron disorders such as spinal muscular atrophy initially present much as the HMSN diseases, but can be distinguished by the lack of sensory findings in SMA. See also *Inherited Causes of Sensorimotor Neuropathy.*

Fenichel (1997).

Peripheral Neuropathy in Patients Referred to a University Clinic

Diagnosis	Percent of Total
Hereditary	29.8
Idiopathic sensory polyneuropathy	23.1
Diabetes mellitus	15.4
Inflammatory demyelinating polyneuropathy	13.1
Multifocal motor neuropathy	5.2
Vitamin B_{12} deficiency	2.2
Idiopathic sensorimotor polyneuropathy with severe distal weakness	1.7
Drug induced	1.5
Sensory neuronopathy	1.0
Other	6.7

Despite the diagnostic tools available, a substantial fraction of patients evaluated for peripheral neuropathy—about 25% in several studies conducted at tertiary referral centers—fall into the "idiopathic" category of causation. Another statistic that emerges from these studies is the large fraction of patients with a hereditary cause of neuropathy. Note that these statistics do not represent the prevalence of neuropathy in the community, where the more common entities are more easily diagnosed. Epidemiological studies have shown that carpal tunnel syndrome is one of the most frequent diagnoses, with a prevalence of about 3% in women (and 0.8% in men). In comparison, the prevalence of hereditary motor and sensory neuropathy (HMSN) is about 20:100,000, and the annual incidence of Guillain-Barré syndrome about 1.7:100,000.

Reprinted with permission from Barohn RJ. Approach to peripheral neuropathy and neuronopathy. *Semin Neurol.* 1998.

Hughes (1995).

Laboratory Testing in Peripheral Neuropathy

Test	Reason
Fasting glucose, CBC, complete serum chemistries, ESR	Metabolic disease such as diabetes, occult alcoholism, vitamin deficiency; vasculitis
Hemoglobin A_1C, glucose tolerance test	Establish level of glycemic control in known diabetic; establish diagnosis in borderline diabetic
Vitamin B_{12}	Pernicious anemia or other cause of B_{12} deficiency
Thyroid function tests	Hypothyroidism
Folate	Rare cause of neuropathy in absence of B_{12} deficiency
Serum protein electrophoresis, serum immunoelectrophoresis	Paraproteinemia, such as multiple myeloma or MGUS, accounts for about 10% of all peripheral neuropathy; SIEP is the more sensitive of the two assays
ANA, RF	SLE, rheumatoid arthritis, Sjögren's syndrome
Anti-MAG antibodies	Subtype of IgM paraproteinemia, associated with a large-fiber sensory neuropathy
Anti-GM1 antibodies	High titers found in 70% of multifocal motor neuropathy (MMN). May also be found in "axonal" GBS
Anti-GQ1b antibodies	Associated with the Miller Fisher variant of GBS
Anti-Hu antibodies	Associated with carcinomatous sensory neuronopathy, often seen in setting of oat cell carcinoma of the lung
Lumbar puncture	Useful in GBS and CIDP to demonstrate diagnostic elevation of CSF protein in absence of significant pleocytosis
Nerve biopsy	Should be considered to establish diagnosis of suspected vasculitis or amyloidosis
Genetic testing	Hereditary motor and sensory neuropathy (HMSN, CMT), hereditary neuropathy with liability to pressure palsy (HNPP)

CIDP: chronic inflammatory demyelinating polyneuropathy; CMT: Charcot-Marie-Tooth disease; GBS: Guillain-Barré syndrome; MGUS: monoclonal gammopathy of undetermined significance; SIEP: serum immunoelectrophoresis.

Griffin et al. (1996).

REFERENCES

Adams RD, Victor M, Ropper AH. *Principles of Neurology.* New York: McGraw-Hill; 1997:1302-1370.

Asbury AK, Tomas PK. The clinical approach to neuropathy. In: Asbury AK, Thomas PK, eds., *Peripheral Nerve Disorders 2.* Oxford: Butterworth-Heinemann; 1995:1–28.

Barohn RJ. Approach to peripheral neuropathy and neuronopathy. *Semin Neurol.* 1998;18:7–18.

Bosch EP, Mitsumoto H. Disorders of peripheral nerves. In: Bradley WG, Daroff RB, Fenichel GM, Marsden CD, eds. *Neurology in Clinical Practice.* 2nd ed. Boston: Butterworth-Heinemann; 1996:1881–1952.

Fenichel GM. *Clinical Pediatric Neurology.* Philadelphia: W.B. Saunders Co.; 1997:176–204.

Griffin JW, Hsieh S-T, McArthur JC, Cornblath DR. Laboratory testing in peripheral nerve disease. *Neurol Clin.* 1996;14:119–133.

Hughes RAC. Epidemiology of peripheral neuropathy. *Curr Opin Neurol.* 1995;8:335–338.

McLeod JG. Invited review: Autonomic dysfunction in peripheral nerve disease. *Muscle Nerve.* 1992;15:3–13.

Poncelet AN. An algorithm for the evaluation of peripheral neuropathy. *Am Fam Physician.* 1998;57:755–764.

Ropper AH, Gorson KC. Neuropathies associated with paraproteinemia. *New Engl J Med.* 1998;338:1601–1607.

Simpson DM, Olney RK. Peripheral neuropathies associated with human immunodeficiency virus infection. *Neurol Clin.* 1992;10:685–709.

Thomas PK, Ochoa J. Clinical features and differential diagnosis. In: Dyck PJ, Thomas PK, eds. *Peripheral Neuropathy.* Philadelphia: W.B. Saunders Co.; 1993:749–774.

10

Infectious Disease

Cheryl A. Jay

Meningitis

	Risk Factors	Onset	Presenting Features	Comments
Acute bacterial meningitis	Extremes of age, head trauma, neurosurgery, craniofacial infection, institutional residence, immune deficiency	Hours to days	Fever, neck stiffness, altered mental status, headache	Triad of fever, neck stiffness, altered mentation seen in ~two-thirds; papilledema rare at presentation; neonates: neck stiffness rare; elderly: features may be subtle; see *Bacterial Meningitis*
Aseptic meningitis	May occur as summer outbreaks	Hours to days	Fever, neck stiffness, headache	Altered mental status or significant cerebral signs incompatible with diagnosis; see *Aseptic Meningitis Syndrome*
Chronic meningitis	Varies	Days to weeks	Headache, fever, neck stiffness, altered mental status	See *Chronic Meningitis*
Subarachnoid hemorrhage	Polycystic kidney disease, HTN; ? oral contraceptives, family history, smoking	Minutes to days	Severe, abrupt headache, sometimes with syncope; neck stiffness; mental status: normal to comatose	Noncontrast CT positive in 90–95%; CSF xanthochromic, bloody

Meningitis usually presents with headache, neck stiffness, and fever. The most frequent causes are shown here. Other infectious considerations include focal bacterial cerebral infections (see *Focal Bacterial Cerebral Infections*), viral encephalitis (see *Viral Encephalitis*), and rickettsial infections. Other noninfectious considerations include neuroleptic malignant syndrome or posterior fossa tumor. See also *CSF Profiles in Meningitis.*

Durand, Calderwood, and Weber (1993); Roos, Tunkel, and Scheld (1997).

Bacterial Meningitis

Patient Group	Likely Pathogens
<3 months	*Streptococcus agalactiae,* *Escherichia coli,* *Listeria monocytogenes*
3 months to <18 years	*Neisseria meningitidis,* *S. pneumoniae,* *Haemophilus influenzae*
18–50 years	*S. pneumoniae,* *N. meningitidis*
>50 years	*S. pneumoniae,* *L. monocytogenes,* gram-negative bacilli
Head trauma, neurosurgery, ventricular shunt	Staphylococci, gram-negative bacilli, *S. pneumoniae*

In 1986, *H. influenzae* was the most common bacterial meningitis pathogen, accounting for 45% of U.S. cases. From 1985 to 1991, the incidence of *H. influenzae* meningitis fell by 82% in children under 5 years of age, related to widespread use of the *H. influenzae* type b vaccine. Another important epidemiologic trend is increasing antibiotic resistance of *S. pneumoniae*. Optimal therapy of meningitis with resistant pneumococcus is uncertain; some strains are resistant not only to penicillin but also commonly used third-generation cephalosporins.

Note that the groups above represent immunocompetent patients; see *CNS Infections in Non-HIV Immunocompromised Patients* for considerations in immunocompromised patients.

Modified with permission from Quagliarello VJ, Scheld WM. Treatment of bacterial meningitis. *New Engl J Med.* 1997.

Aseptic Meningitis Syndrome

	Common	*Uncommon*	*Other Considerations*
Viral	Enteroviruses, arbo-viruses, HSV-2	Mumps, human herpes virus 6, lymphocytic choriomeningitis virus, human immu-nodeficiency virus	Other herpesviruses (HSV-1, VZV, CMV, EBV), influenza A and B, measles, rotavirus, coronavirus, enceph-alomyocarditis virus, parvovirus 19, among many others
Bacterial	*Borrelia burgdorferi* (Lyme disease), par-tially treated bacte-rial meningitis (with common pathogens), parameningeal in-fection	*Mycobacterium tuber-culosis, Leptospira* spp.	*Brucella* spp., *Myco-plasma hominis, M. pneumoniae*
Fungal		*Cryptococcus neofor-mans, Coccidiodes immitis, Histo-plasma capsulatum, Candida* spp., *Blas-tomyces dermatitidis*	Many others
Other			*Toxoplasma gondii,* autoimmune disor-ders, Behçet's syn-drome, drugs (sulfa, NSAIDs, immuno-modulators, among others), neoplasms

HSV-1: herpes simplex virus type 1; HSV-2: herpes simplex virus type 2; VZV: varicella-zoster virus; CMV: cytomegalovirus; EBV: Epstein-Barr virus.

Aseptic meningitis is defined as a meningeal inflammatory clinical syndrome in which common bacterial pathogens cannot be identified. This implies a self-limited illness and absence of symptoms or signs of parenchymal brain dysfunction (which would signify encephalitis) or spinal cord involvement (which would indicate myelitis). Most cases are caused by viruses, but other nonviral pathogens and noninfectious disorders may also cause the syndrome. See also *CSF Findings in Bacterial vs. Aseptic Meningitis.*

Rotbart (1997).

CSF Findings in Bacterial vs. Aseptic Meningitis

	Bacterial Meningitis	*Aseptic Meningitis*
Opening pressure	Elevated (>180 mm water)	Normal or slightly elevated
Protein	Increased (often >100 mg/dL)	Normal or increased
Glucose	Decreased (<40 mg/dL)	Normal (>45 mg/dL)
CSF-serum glucose ratio	<0.3	>0.6
White blood cell count	Increased (often >1,000/mm^3, neutrophil predominance)	Increased (10–2,000/mm^3, lymphocyte predominance)
Gram stain	Positive in 50–80% of untreated patients	Negative
Culture	Positive in 85% of untreated patients	Negative

Blood cultures may be positive even when CSF culture is negative and should be obtained in all patients with suspected bacterial meningitis, prior to administering antibiotics. CSF antigen-detection tests for common bacterial pathogens are highly specific but not sensitive and should not be used to exclude the diagnosis of bacterial meningitis. See also *Meningitis* and *Aseptic Meningitis Syndrome*.

Modified with permission from Phillips EJ, Simor AE. Bacterial meningitis in children and adults: Changes in community-acquired disease may affect patient care. *Postgrad Med.* 1998.

Chronic Meningitis

	Cause	Comment
Infectious/parainfectious		
Bacterial	*Mycobacterium tuberculosis*	See *Neurotuberculosis*
	Treponema pallidum (syphilis)	See *Neurosyphilis*
	Borrelia burgdorferi (Lyme disease)	Endemic to northeastern, upper midwestern, and Pacific coastal United States; Europe
Fungal	*Cryptococcus neoformans*	CSF cryptococcal antigen >90% sensitive
	Coccidiodes immitis	Endemic to southwestern United States, Central and South America
	Histoplasma capsulatum	Endemic to Ohio, central Mississippi Valley, Appalachia region
Parainfectious	Partially treated bacterial meningitis	
	Parameningeal infection	Adjacent craniofacial or paraspinal infection
	Endocarditis or bacteremia	
Noninfectious		
	Sarcoidosis	Cranial neuropathies, hypothalamic dysfunction (especially diabetes insipidus) often associated
	Leptomeningeal metastases	Fever, meningismus less prominent than in infectious etiologies; cerebral, cranial nerve, spinal root deficits common
	Vasculitis: granulomatous angiitis, SLE	
	Drugs	NSAIDs, sulfa, IVIG, and other immune modulators, others
	Behçet's disease	Recurrent oral and genital ulcers, uveitis, skin lesions

Chronic meningitis is characterized by subacute headache, fever, and stiff neck, often with evidence of parenchymal dysfunction, and is accompanied by abnormal CSF (elevated protein, normal or moderately low glucose, lymphocytic pleocytosis). Some authorities require the syndrome to be present for 4 weeks; most patients require evaluation prior to this.

Other infectious causes: other bacteria (Actinomyces, *Listeria monocytogenes, Nocardia asteroides*), other fungi, parasites, viruses (enterovirus in immunosuppressed patients, HIV), among many others.

Other noninfectious causes: Vogt-Koyanagi-Harada syndrome, unrecognized subarachnoid hemorrhage, other vasculitides, CNS tumors (epidermoid, glioma, craniopharyngioma), migraine, seizure, idiopathic.

Gripshover and Ellner (1997).

CSF Profiles in Meningitis

Pathogen	White Blood Cell Count	Predominant Cell	Glucose	Protein
Common bacteria	100s–1,000s	Neutrophil	Decreased	Elevated
Viruses (includes Mollaret's)	10s–100s	Mononuclear	Normal or slightly decreased	Normal or slightly elevated
Leptospira, Lyme, myco-plasma				
Parameningeal infection, partially treated bacterial meningitis				
Mycobacterial, Brucella, fungal, toxoplasma	10s–100s	Mononuclear	Decreased	Elevated
Autoimmune disorders	10s–100s	Neutrophil	Normal or slightly decreased	Normal or slightly elevated
Parameningeal infection, partially treated bacterial meningitis				

Note that, in parameningeal infection or partially treated meningitis, either of the two patterns shown may be seen. In toxoplasma infection, glucose usually is normal.

Rotbart (1997).

Focal Bacterial Cerebral Infections

	Risk Factors	Onset	Presenting Features	Comments
Brain abscess	Craniofacial infection, head trauma or neurosurgery, hematogenous, immune compromise	Varies	Headache, focal deficit; fever in ~50%	Hematogenous sources: congenital heart disease, chronic lung infection, endocarditis Papilledema in ~25% CT/MRI: cerebritis or ring-enhancing lesion(s) Pathogens listed in *Brain Abscess* (next)
Subdural empyema	Craniofacial infection, head trauma or neurosurgery, hematogenous	Acute	Fever, headache, focal deficit, altered consciousness, neck stiffness	Predominant predisposing cause: sinusitis Papilledema in ~33%; CT features often subtle early; MRI preferred Common pathogens: *Streptococcus* spp., *Staphylococcus* spp., other anaerobes, gram-negative bacilli May complicate meningitis in neonates
Epidural abscess	Craniotomy, craniofacial infection	Varies	Fever, headache, local skull tenderness	Focal deficit, altered consciousness, seizures may develop later in course; CT/MRI: enhancing lentiform extra-axial collection; common pathogens: *Streptococcus* spp., *Staphylococcus* spp., other anaerobes

Lumbar puncture usually is contraindicated and rarely yields causative organism(s), unless there is concomitant meningitis. Given common risk factors, these disorders may develop in combination with each other or with bacterial meningitis.

Gellin, Weingarten, and Gamache (1997); Helfgott, Weingarten, and Harman (1997); Wispelwey, Darcy, and Scheld (1997).

Brain Abscess

Source	Site	Pathogens
Paranasal sinus	Frontal lobe	Aerobic and anaerobic streptococci, *Haemophilus* spp., *Bacteroides* spp. (non-*fragilis*), *Fusobacterium* spp.
Ear infection	Temporal lobe, cerebellum	*Streptococcus* spp. Enterobacteriaceae *Bacteroides* spp. (including *fragilis*)
Hematogenous	Multiple, often in middle cerebral artery distribution	Depends on source: endocarditis (*Staphylococcus aureus*, Viridans streptococci); urinary tract (Enterobacteriaceae, Pseudomonaceae); intraabdominal (*Streptococcus* spp., Enterobacteriaceae, anaerobes); lung abscess (*Streptococcus* spp., *Actinomyces* spp., *Fusobacterium* spp.)
Trauma	Depends on wound site	*S. aureus*, *Clostridium* spp., Enterobacteriaceae
Postoperative	Depends on wound site	*S. epidermidis*, *S. aureus*, Enterobacteriaceae, Pseudomonaceae

Brain abscess is uncommon in neonates but should be considered in meningitis or bacteremia due to *Citrobacter diversus*, *Proteus* spp., *Serratia marcescens*, or *Enterobacter spp*. In children, cyanotic congenital heart disease is a common predisposing factor. Modern therapy of ear infections has decreased the incidence of otogenic brain abscess in developed nations. Fungal or parasitic abscesses occur in patients from endemic areas, or with immune deficiency. See *CNS Complications of HIV Infection* for considerations in AIDS patients, and *CNS Infections in Non-HIV Immunocompromised Patients* for considerations in other immunocompromised patients.

Modified with permission from Mathisen GE, Johnson JP. Brain abscess. *Clin Infect Dis.* 1997.

Viral Encephalitis

Presenting features	Fever, headache, parenchymal cerebral dysfunction (altered consciousness, focal signs, seizures)
	Nuchal rigidity if meningoencephalitis, cord signs if encephalomyelitis
Pathogens	Arboviruses: St. Louis, eastern equine, western equine, California encephalitis viruses, among others (United States); Japanese encephalitis (Asia)
	HSV (type 1 in adults, type 2 in neonates): 10% of U.S. encephalitis cases
	Other herpesviruses: EBV, CMV, HHV-6
	Enteroviruses: coxsackievirus, echovirus (more commonly cause aseptic meningitis)
	Rabies: uniformly fatal, once established
	Others: adenovirus, LCM, paramyxoviruses (mumps, measles), HIV
Historical clues	Arboviruses in tick and mosquito season, enteroviruses in late summer and fall, LCM in winter
	Enterovirus encephalitis may occur as family outbreaks
	Travel: exposure to other arboviruses and unusual pathogens
	Dog, cat, bat, or wild carnivore exposure in rabies; rodents in LCM
Differential diagnosis	Other CNS infections: bacterial (including abscess), tubercular, rickettsial, fungal, parasitic
	Postinfectious encephalomyelitis
	Noninfectious: stroke, tumor, toxic encephalopathy, subdural hematoma, adrenoleukodystrophy, Reye's syndrome, vasculitis
Diagnostic studies	CT/MRI: excludes other diagnoses; reveals temporal and orbitofrontal abnormalities in HSV encephalitis
	CSF: elevated protein, mononuclear pleocytosis; in HSV, may see RBCs, xanthochromia; HSV PCR sensitive and specific; viral culture or serologic testing helpful in some circumstances
	EEG: periodic epileptiform discharges in HSV encephalitis
	Serologic evaluation: acute and convalescent titers

HSV: herpes simplex virus; EBV: Epstein-Barr virus; CMV: cytomegalovirus; HHV-6: human herpesvirus 6; LCM: lymphocytic choriomeningitis virus.

Neuroimaging, CSF, and EEG assist in establishing diagnosis of viral encephalitis. Identifying specific viral pathogens with serologic testing rarely influences therapy but assists in public health surveillance and prognosis, as outcome varies by viral pathogen. HSV encephalitis and eastern equine encephalitis have high mortality rates, with significant neurologic sequelae in survivors. HSV encephalitis is the major treatable encephalitis in the United States, and it is customary to empirically administer high-dose intravenous acyclovir to all patients with suspected viral encephalitis.

Johnson (1996); Whitley et al. (1989).

Neurologic Complications of Infective Endocarditis

Syndrome	*Mechanism*
Stroke	
Ischemic	Septic emboli with infarction
Parenchymal hemorrhage	Hemorrhagic infarction or mycotic aneurysm, rupture
Subarachnoid hemorrhage	Mycotic aneurysm rupture
Acute encephalopathy	Microemboli or microabscesses
Meningitis	Bacteremia, with meningeal seeding, microabscesses, ruptured macroabscess
Brain abscess	Bacteremia
Myelopathy	Diskitis or vertebral osteomyelitis, septic emboli with infarction (rare)

Neurologic complications develop in about one-third of patients with endocarditis, and constitute the presenting feature in up to one-fourth. Seizures may occur as a consequence of cerebral complications or associated toxic-metabolic states. Headache likewise may indicate any of the above cerebral complications but has also been described as an initial symptom leading to diagnosis of endocarditis. In addition to bacterial meningitis, the aseptic meningitis syndrome may be seen.

Other complications include: visual disturbance due to retinal emboli or cranial nerve dysfunction, mononeuropathy from emboli.

Francioli (1997); Jones and Siekert (1989).

Spinal Epidural Abscess

Presenting features	Fever, back pain (and tenderness), radiculopathy, progressive myelopathy
Source	Contiguous infection: vertebral osteomyelitis; retroperitoneal, perinephric, or psoas abscess; decubitus ulcer, dermal sinus tract, spinal surgery or procedures (including LP, epidural catheters) Hematogenous infection: injection drug use, endocarditis, skin or soft tissue infection None identified in 30%
Location	Cervical: 21%; thoracic: 44%; lumbosacral: 35%
Systemic misdiagnoses	Musculoskeletal pain, disk disease, arthritis, urinary tract infection, endocarditis, acute abdomen, viral syndrome, fibrositis, myocardial infarction, prostate disease, drug fever, pregnancy
Neurologic misdiagnoses	Spinal TB, meningitis, zoster, infectious polyneuritis, transverse myelitis, Guillain-Barré syndrome, spinal cord hematoma or tumor, stroke, poliomyelitis, hysteria, epidural lipomatosis
Pathogens	*Staphylococcus aureus,* gram-negative bacilli Others: *S. epidermidis*, aerobic streptococci, anaerobes, fungi *Mycobacterium tuberculosis* accounts for up to 25% of cases in some series

The combination of back pain, local tenderness, and fever always should suggest the possibility of spinal epidural abscess, a neurologic emergency. Abscess cultures reveal the organism in 90% of causes; blood cultures are positive in 62%. Plain films may reveal disk or bony changes that suggest the diagnosis, but normal results do not exclude the diagnosis. MRI or CT myelography are the preferred imaging studies. LP usually is contraindicated due to risk of spinal herniation and, for lumbosacral abscesses, risk of seeding the subarachnoid space. CSF cultures usually do not reveal the causative organism. Most cases require emergent neurosurgical intervention, as prognosis depends on severity and duration of neurologic dysfunction at time of surgery. Other infectious causes of myelopathy: other bacteria (syphilis, Lyme), viruses (HTLV-1, HIV, herpesviruses), parasites, postinfectious, or postvaccinial.

Gellin et al. (1997).

Neurotuberculosis

	Presenting Features	Studies	Complications	Comments
TB meningitis	Fever, headache, nausea, vomiting, altered mental status; also cranial neuropathy, ischemic stroke	CSF: high protein, low glucose, lymphocytic pleocytosis; AFB smear positive ~25%, culture positive ~25% CXR**: 50–90% children, 25–50% adults PPD positive: 85–90% of children, 40–65% of adults	Hydrocephalus ischemic stroke, SIADH, radiculomyelitis*	Prior TB history: 55% children, 8-12% adults Higher yield of AFB smear and culture with repeated high-volume LPs Cultures grow slowly; treatment usually empiric Consider in all cases of chronic meningitis and suspected bacterial meningitis failing antibacterial therapy
Pott's disease	Subacute or chronic back pain, para- or quadriparesis	Plain spine films, MRI or CT-myelogram	Gibbus, spinal instability	Accounts for up to 25% of spinal epidural infections in some series
Tuberculoma	Progressive focal cerebral or spinal cord dysfunction	Contrast-enhanced CT or MRI		Rare

*May antecede typical TB meningitis or occur in the absence of intracranial disease ("spinal meningitis"). **Abnormalities compatible with remote or current TB. SIADH: syndrome of inappropriate antidiuretic hormone secretion; PPD: purified protein derivative.

Lymphocytic meningitis, with elevated protein and low glucose, always should raise the suspicion of TB meningitis. In the United States, TB cases have been increasing, in part due to the AIDS epidemic. Extrapulmonary TB, including CNS disease, is more common in HIV-infected patients. Tuberculous abscess is rare and refers to a tuberculoma with a liquified core. The course is more rapid, and patients appear more acutely ill.

Zuger and Lowy (1997).

Neurosyphilis

	Onset	Early Clinical Features	Later Manifestations	Comments
Acute syphilitic meningitis	2 yr	Headache, stiff neck, nausea, vomiting	Cranial neuropathies, hydrocephalus	Patients often afebrile
Meningovascular syphilis	4–7 years	Subacute prodrome: headache, vertigo, personality change, insomnia, seizure, TIA	Focal cerebral ischemia	
Parenchymal forms				
General paresis	10–20 years	Impaired memory, personality, and mood changes	Psychosis, tremor, seizures	
Tabes dorsalis	15–20 years	Lightning pains, paresthesias, pupillary changes, hyporeflexia	Bladder dysfunction, sensory ataxia, Charcot's joints	CSF may be less abnormal than in paretic and meningeal forms
Gummatous	Any time	Progressive focal cerebral or cord dysfunction		Rare
Asymptomatic	Any time	None (defined as abnormal CSF with normal neurologic exam)	None	CNS invasion common in early syphilis

Time of onset shown is after primary infection. The Centers for Disease Control recommend LP for syphilis patients who have neurologic or ophthalmic signs or symptoms, evidence of active tertiary disease (aortitis, gumma, iritis), treatment failure, HIV infection with late latent syphilis, or syphilis of unknown duration.

Accepted sensitivity of CSF serology for diagnosis of neurosyphilis is 30–70%. CSF-VDRL is highly specific, establishing the diagnosis if CSF is not bloody. Otherwise, the diagnosis rests on clinical findings, serum serology, and CSF protein and cell count, even if CSF-VDRL is negative. CSF-FTA is not specific but is believed to be highly sensitive; some authorities suggest that a negative result excludes neurosyphilis.

Centers for Disease Control (1998); Hook and Marra (1992); Simon (1985).

CNS Complications of HIV Infection

Syndrome	Common Causes	CD4	Studies	Comments
Focal cerebral dysfunction	Toxoplasmosis	<200	Serum toxoplasma serology; CT/MRI: enhancing lesion(s)	Acute to subacute, often with fever or headache
	PML	<100	CT/MRI: nonenhancing white matter lesion(s)	Usually subacute
	PCNSL	<100	CT/MRI: enhancing lesion(s)	Usually subacute
Diffuse cerebral dysfunction	HIV dementia	<200	MRI: atrophy; symmetric, ill-defined white matter abnormalities	Behavioral, cognitive, motor slowing; early in course, resembles depression
	CMV encephalitis	<50	CT/MRI: periventricular enhancement CSF profile may resemble bacterial meningitis, with positive CMV PCR	Rapidly progressive confusion, sometimes with prominent brainstem dysfunction, hydrocephalus, or hyponatremia
Meningitis	Cryptococcal meningitis	<200	CSF: routine studies may be nonspecific; cryptococcal antigen >90% sensitive	Meningeal signs and symptoms often minimal
	HIV-related	Any	CSF: mild protein elevation, lymphocytic pleocytosis	Aseptic (monophasic or recurrent) and chronic forms seen; asymptomatic CSF abnormalities much more common
Myelopathy	HIV myelopathy	<200	MRI: negative	Subacute to chronic; pathologically and clinically similar to B$_{12}$ deficiency
	Herpesviruses (VZV, CMV, HSV)	<200	MRI: cord swelling, enhancement; viral PCR in CSF may be helpful	Acute to subacute

PML: progressive multifocal leukoencephalopathy; PCNSL: primary CNS lymphoma; CMV: cytomegalovirus; PCR: polymerase chain reaction; VZV: varicella-zoster virus; HSV: herpes simplex virus.

Price (1996); Simpson and Tagliati (1994).

Neuromuscular Complications of HIV Infection

Syndrome	Common Causes	CD4	Studies	Comments
Neuropathic pain	HIV neuropathy	<200	EMG/NCS: distal axonopathy	Length dependent, often painful poly-neuropathy; typically diagnosed clinically
	Nucleoside neuropathy	Any	EMG/NCS: distal axonopathy	Resembles HIV neuropathy clinically; dose-limiting toxicity of ddI, ddC, d4T
Neuropathy with weakness	Demyelinating	>500	EMG/NCS: demyelination CSF: elevated protein, lymphocytic pleocytosis	Acute and chronic forms, clinically similar to syndromes in seronegative patients, except for pleocytosis
	Mononeuritis multiplex	>500	EMG/NCS: multifocal abnormalities	Often self-limited
		<50	EMG/NCS: multifocal abnormalities	Often progressive and due to CMV
	Polyradiculopathy	<50	CSF: profile resembles bacterial meningitis; CMV PCR positive	Clinical features suggest cauda equina syndrome
Myopathy	HIV related	Any	Elevated serum CK EMG/NCS: inflammatory myopathy Biopsy: inflammatory myopathy	Resembles polymyositis clinically and histologically
	Zidovudine	Any	Elevated serum CK Biopsy: mitochondrial abnormalities	Clinically similar to HIV-related myopathy; occurs after >6 mon therapy

ddI: didanosine; ddC: zalcitabine; d4T: stavudine; CMV: cytomegalovirus; PCR: polymerase chain reaction.

For neuropathic pain in HIV-positive patients, also consider exposure to isoniazid, dapsone, or ethanol; diabetes; B$_{12}$ deficiency. Some neuromuscular syndromes may be seen in patients not known to be HIV positive. See also *Peripheral Neuropathy in Patients with HIV Infection*, in Chapter 9.

Price (1996); Simpson and Tagliati (1994).

CNS Infections in Non-HIV Immunocompromised Patients

	Impaired Cell-Mediated Immunity	Inadequate Neutrophil Number or Function
Clinical settings	Lymphoma, organ transplant recipients, chronic corticosteroid therapy, HIV infection	Acute leukemia, aplastic anemia, cytotoxic chemotherapy
Acute meningitis	Listeria monocytogenes	Pseudomonas aeruginosa, Enterobacteriaceae, also Candida spp.
Subacute or chronic meningitis	Cryptococcus neoformans; Mycobacteria tuberculosis; also L. monocytogenes, Strongyloides stercoralis, atypical mycobacteria, Coccidiodes immitis	Candida spp.
Meningoencephalitis	L. monocytogenes; Toxoplasma gondii; Varicella-zoster virus; also progressive multifocal leukoencephalopathy, S. stercoralis, C. neoformans	P. aeruginosa, Candida spp., Enterobacteriaceae
Brain abscess	Aspergillus spp.; Nocardia asteroides; T. gondii; also C. neoformans, L. monocytogenes, Mucorales	Aspergillus spp.; mucorales; Candida spp.; also P. aeruginosa, Enterobacteriaceae

Impaired immunity from any cause increases the risk of CNS infection. Symptoms and signs may be less dramatic than those in immunocompetent patients. Given the high risk and subtle clinical features, a low threshold should be maintained for evaluating immunocompromised patients for CNS infection. Patients with defective humoral immunity (chronic lymphocytic leukemia, multiple myeloma, or Hodgkin's disease following chemotherapy and radiotherapy) or who are asplenic (trauma, sickle cell disease, among others) are at increased risk for meningitis due to encapsulated organisms (*Streptococcus pneumoniae*, *Haemophilus influenzae*, and less commonly, *Neisseria meningitidis*). Note that the spectrum of CNS infections in HIV-infected patients (see *CNS Complications of HIV Infection*) overlaps with, but is not identical to, patients with impaired cell-mediated immunity from other causes.

Rubin and Hooper (1985).

REFERENCES

Centers for Disease Control and Prevention. 1998 guidelines for treatment of sexually transmitted diseases. *MMWR*. 1998;47:35.

Durand ML, Calderwood SB, Weber DJ, et al. Acute bacterial meningitis in adults: A review of 493 episodes. *New Engl J Med*. 1993;328:21–28.

Francioli PB. Complications of infective endocarditis. In: Scheld WM, Whitley RJ, Durack DT, eds. *Infections of the Central Nervous System*. Philadelphia: Lippincott-Raven; 1997:523–53.

Gellin BG, Weingarten K, Gamache Jr FW, Hartman BJ. Epidural abscess. In: Scheld WM, Whitley RJ, Durack DT, eds. *Infections of the Central Nervous System*. Philadelphia: Lippincott-Raven; 1997:507–522.

Gripshover BM, Ellner JJ. Chronic meningitis syndrome and meningitis of noninfective or uncertain etiology. In: Scheld WM, Whitley RJ, Durack DT, eds. *Infections of the Central Nervous System*. Philadelphia: Lippincott-Raven; 1997:881–896.

Helfgott DC, Weingarten K, Harman BJ. Subdural empyema. In: Scheld WM, Whitley RJ, Durack DT, (eds). *Infectious of the Central Nervous System*. Philadelphia: Lippincott-Raven; 1997:495-505.

Hook EW, Marra CM. Acquired syphilis in adults. *New Engl J Med*. 1992; 326:1060–1069.

Johnson RT. Acute encephalitis. *Clin Infect Dis*. 1996;23:219–226.

Jones HR, Siekert RG. Neurologic manifestations of infective endocarditis: Review of clinical and therapeutic challenges. *Brain*. 1989;112:1295–1315.

Mathisen GE, Johnson JP. Brain abscess. *Clin Infect Dis*. 1997;25:763–781.

Phillips EJ, Simor AE. Bacterial meningitis in children and adults: Changes in community-acquired disease may affect patient care. *Postgrad Med*. 1998;103:102–117.

Price RW. Neurological complications of HIV infection. *Lancet*. 1996; 348:445–452.

Quagliarello VJ, Scheld WM. Treatment of bacterial meningitis. *New Engl J Med*. 1997;336:708–716.

Roos KL, Tunkel AR, Scheld WM. Acute bacterial meningitis in children and adults. In: Scheld WM, Whitley RJ, Durack DT, eds. *Infections of the Central Nervous System*. Philadelphia: Lippincott-Raven; 1997:335–401.

Rotbart HA. Viral meningitis and the aseptic meningitis syndrome. In: Scheld WM, Whitley RJ, Durack DT, eds. *Infections of the Central Nervous System*. Philadelphia: Lippincott-Raven: 1997:23–46.

Rubin RH, Hooper DC. Central nervous system infection in the compromised host. *Med Clin N Am*. 1985;69:281–296.

Simon RF. Neurosyphilis. *Arch Neurol*. 1985;42:606–613.

Simpson DM, Tagliati M. Neurologic manifestations of HIV infection. *Ann Int Med*. 1994;121:769–785.

Whitley RJ, Cobbs CG, Alford CA, et al. Diseases that mimic herpes simplex encephalitis: Diagnosis, presentation and outcome. *JAMA*. 1989; 262:234–239.

Wispelwey B, Dacey RG, Scheld WM. Brain abscess. In: Scheld WM, Whitley RJ, Durack DT, eds. *Infections of the Central Nervous System.* Philadelphia: Lippincott-Raven; 1997:463–493.

Zuger A, Lowy FD. Tuberculosis. In: Scheld WM, Whitley RJ, Durack DT, eds. *Infections of the Central Nervous System.* Philadelphia: Lippincott-Raven; 1997:417–443.

11

Behavioral Neurology

George M. Ringholz

Left Hemisphere Disorders: Alexia, Dyslexia, and Apraxia

Syndrome	Features	Localization
Alexia with agraphia	Cannot read or write (not aided by spelling words aloud)	Left angular gyrus or left posterior inferior temporal lobe
Alexia without agraphia	Can write but not read; aided by spelling words aloud	Medial left occipital cortex *and* splenium of corpus callosum; or left lateral geniculate body *and* splenium of corpus callosum
Deep dyslexia	Makes semantic errors; concrete words easier; difficulty with functors (articles and pronouns); unable to read nonwords	Large perisylvian lesions, associated with aphasia
Phonologic dyslexia	Reading without print-to-sound conversion, impaired reading of nonword letter strings	Dominant perisylvian cortex superior temporal lobe, angular gyrus
Surface dyslexia	Inability to pronounce words of nonphonologic pronunciation (e.g., cough, rough, bough)	Alzheimer's disease; poorly localized
Ideomotor apraxia	Inability to perform learned movements to command, not accounted for by deficits in strength, sensation, coordination, or comprehension	Left inferior parietal lobe, arcuate fasciculus
Limb-kinetic apraxia	Loss of dexterity and coordination of distal limb movements not accounted for by weakness or sensory loss	Supplementary motor cortex contralateral to deficit
Sympathetic apraxia	Ideomotor apraxia of left hand, with right hemiparesis and Broca's aphasia	Left frontal lobe
Callosal apraxia	Rare condition of ideomotor apraxia of left hand, without hemiparesis or aphasia	Anterior callosal fibers
Ideational apraxia	Inability to perform a sequence of learned acts (multistep)	Diffuse brain injury, dementia

Alexia, agraphia, and apraxia typically are associated with left hemisphere dysfunction. Alexia is the acquired inability to read, which may occur with or without agraphia, the acquired inability to write. Although uncommon, alexia without agraphia is a striking syndrome that results from two separate lesions, one that damages visual processing in the dominant (language-producing) hemisphere and one that prevents the transfer of visual information from the nondominant hemisphere. Apraxia is the inability to carry out skilled motor activities to verbal command, despite intact motor and sensory function. Left-handers are right hemisphere dominant for praxis.

Benson (1993); Heilman and Rothi (1993).

Right Hemisphere Disorders: Neglect, Anosognosia, and Constructional Apraxia

Syndrome	Features	Localization
Unilateral neglect	Lack of attention to events and actions in one-half of space; can involve all sensory modalities, as well as motor acts and motivation	Left or right parietal lesions or subcortical; most severe and persistent in right parietal damage
Anosognosia	Denial of hemiparesis or other disability Risk factors include left-neglect, other cognitive deficits, apathy	Large right-sided lesions
Tactile agnosia	Impaired unilateral tactile object recognition	Inferior parietal cortex; contralateral, lateral somatosensory association cortex
Astereognosis	Impaired tactile perception	Somatosensory pathways; right hemisphere
Facial discrimination	Inability to discriminate nonfamiliar faces	Right temporal lobe lesions
Dressing "apraxia"	Body-garment disorientation, unilateral neglect	Right parietal lesions
Constructional "apraxia"	Inability to copy, model, or construct complex figures	May be caused by occipital, frontal, or parietal lesions in either hemisphere; most severe with right parietal damage
Topographical disorientation	Inability to find one's way in a familiar environment or learn new paths.	Right parietal lobe; often seen in dementia
Reduplicative amnesia	Recognize immediate surroundings but believe they are in a different location	Right frontal and parietal lesions, often seen in Alzheimer's disease
Executive aprosodia	Speech is monotonous, unable to convey emotion	Lateral inferior frontal lobe; is right hemisphere equivalent of Broca's area
Receptive aprosodia	Unable to comprehend emotional and tonal aspects of communication	Right posterior, superior temporal lobe; is right hemisphere equivalent of Wernicke's area

Agnosia is the inability to recognize common objects, despite intact primary sensory function. Aprosodia is the right hemisphere counterpart of aphasia and consists of the loss of the "musical" components of language, such as tone of voice.

Constructional and dressing "apraxias" may not be true apraxias, that is, syndromes of loss of skilled movements; rather, they probably represent complex deficits of higher motor and sensory processing that lead to loss of specific abilities.

Benton and Tranel (1993); Heilman, Watson, and Valenstein (1993); Mesulam (1981).

Aphasia

Syndrome	Fluency	Comprehension	Repetition	Localization
Wernicke's	Fluent	Impaired	Impaired	Posterior, superior temporal lobe
Transcortical sensory	Fluent	Impaired	Intact	Angular gyrus
Conduction	Fluent	Intact	Impaired	Arcuate fasciculus
Anomic	Fluent	Intact	Intact	Anterior temporal angular gyrus
Broca's	Nonfluent	Intact	Impaired	Inferior frontal
Transcortical motor	Nonfluent	Intact	Intact	Medial frontal lobe, superior to Broca's area
Global	Nonfluent	Impaired	Impaired	Sum of Broca's and Wernicke's
Mixed transcortical	Nonfluent	Impaired	Intact	Sum of transcortical motor and transcortical sensory

Aphasia is the acquired loss of language. Aphasia may be classified according to whether the production of language (whether spoken, written, or by some other means) is fluent or nonfluent, whether comprehension of language is intact or impaired, and whether the ability to repeat is intact or impaired. The most basic distinction concerns fluency, with fluent aphasias characterized by normal or increased rate of spontaneous speech, preserved speech melody, normal phrase length, and preserved grammatical constructions but also marked by empty speech with poor information content and frequent paraphasic errors. Nonfluent aphasias, on the other hand, show sparse, effortful verbal output with short phrase length, abnormal prosody, and agrammatism; these may be associated with dysarthria.

Note that 99% of right-handers have left hemisphere–dominant language; of left-handers, 70% also are left hemisphere dominant, 15% are bilateral, and 15% are right hemisphere dominant.

Cummings and Trimble (1995:76).

Altered Perception

Syndrome	Features	Localization
Visual object agnosia	Inability to recognize common objects	Bilateral medial occipito-temporal lesions
Achromatopsia	Central color blindness in contralateral visual field	Medial occipital lobe inferior to calcarine fissure
Cortical blindness	May be totally blind, able to count fingers, or have light perception only; may have macular sparing; may be associated with Anton's syndrome	Bilateral optic radiations or occipital cortex
Simultanagnosia	Inability to perceive more than one part of the visual field at a time; may be associated with Balint's syndrome	Bilateral parieto-occipital junction
Prosopagnosia	Inability to recognize familiar faces, despite normal sight and facial discrimination	Bilateral occipito-temporal lesions
Cortical deafness	Inability to compare and contrast different sounds; deficits in speech comprehension, speech repetition, musical perception, recognition of familiar sounds, musical perception, vocal prosody	Bilateral Heschl's gyrus
Pure word deafness	Disorder of speech comprehension, speech repetition, and musical perception	Bilateral anterior superior temporal gyrus
Auditory sound agnosia	Disorder of recognition of familiar sounds, musical perception	Temporoparietal junction

See also *Neurobehavioral Syndromes.*

Damasio (1985).

Memory Loss

Syndrome	Cause	Features
Dementia	Alzheimer's disease	Memory impairment often is the earliest sign, followed by deficits in orientation, judgment, memory, and abstract thinking.
	Frontotemporal lobar degeneration	Memory disorders often occur late, are associated with poor insight and interference effects (learning of new information "erases" older information).
	Parkinson's disease	Slowing of thought and motor performance with associated memory impairment.
Wernicke-Korsakoff syndrome	Thiamine deficiency due to chronic alcohol abuse, stomach cancer, or severe malnutrition	Wernicke's encephalopathy: oculomotor disturbance, gait ataxia, and confusion. Korsakoff's psychosis: severe amnesia with confabulation, personality changes, and frontal lobe signs.
Traumatic brain injury	Structural damage to frontal and anterior temporal lobes, diffuse axonal injury, hypoxia.	Acute: posttraumatic amnesia, confusion, and disorientation. Chronic: deficits in both new learning and retrieval.
Temporal lobe surgery	Bilateral temporal lobectomy Left temporal lobectomy Right temporal lobectomy	Severe global amnesia. Impairment of verbal memory and naming. Impairment in memory for geometric shapes, tones, faces.
Encephalitis	Herpes simplex, herpes zoster, postinfection with influenza: primarily involves temporal lobes and orbitofrontal areas	Acute: headache, vomiting, irritability, delirium, seizures. Chronic: severe antero- and retrograde amnesia.
Vascular amnesias	Posterior cerebral artery infarction Anterior communicating artery aneurysm	Loss of new learning, visual field defects. Deficits in temporal ordering and contextual learning. Retrieval poor, with relative sparing of new learning.
Transient global amnesia	Thalamic or bilateral temporal ischemia due to migraine, seizures, or posterior circulation insufficiency	Sudden onset of anterograde amnesia, usually lasting several hours with complete recovery. Insight remains good even during the attack. Speech is unimpaired.

Other causes of amnestic syndromes include cerebral anoxia due to cardiac arrest, cyanide poisoning, or complications of general anesthesia; electro-convulsive therapy; carbon monoxide poisoning; malnutrition; hypoglycemia; and the pseudodementia of depression.

Wilson (1987).

Hallucination and Illusion

Syndrome	Features	Localization or Cause
Visual hallucinations	May be flashes of light, colors, shapes, or formed objects depending on lesion site	Lesions anywhere in visual pathways, from eyes to occipital cortex
	"Fortifications" or "scintillating scotomas" may precede migraines	Occipital cortex
	Colored shapes, especially circular, may occur in occipital epilepsy	Occipital cortex
	Complex visual hallucinations seen with drug intoxication or other causes of delirium, and dementia with Lewy bodies	Diffuse
Auditory hallucinations	May be clicks, sounds, voices	Acquired deafness, brainstem lesions, temporal lobe seizures, psychosis
Gustatory/ olfactory hallucinations	Unpleasant tastes and/or smells, such as "burning rubber"	Associated with temporal lobe seizures
Dysmnestic hallucinations	Déjà vu (false sense of familiarity of a situation) or jamais vu (false sense of novelty of a situation)	Associated with temporal lobe seizures
Peduncular hallucinations	Sleep disturbance and Lilliputian hallucinations (visions of "little people")	Associated with midbrain lesions
Formicative hallucinations	Feeling that insects are crawling on the skin	Usually a result of drug intoxication
Hypnagogic/ hypnopompic hallucinations	Auditory, visual or tactile hallucination while falling asleep or on awakening, respectively	Seen as part of narcolepsy syndrome
Visual illusions	Macropsia/micropsia (distortion of size and distance of seen objects)	Associated with temporal lobe seizures
	Palinopsia (persistent afterimages)	Metabolic disorders, drugs, occipital epilepsy
	Polyopia (multiple images of single object)	Refractive error in eye; occipital cortex

Hallucination is perception without primary sensory input. Illusion is a distortion of sensory input. While hallucinations are a common feature of both neurologic (e.g., epilepsy) and psychiatric disease (e.g., schizophrenia), neurologic causes of hallucination are more likely to result in "unformed" sensations (i.e., elementary shapes and sounds) and, with an ictal cause, are usually stereotyped. "Formed" hallucinations, such as voices speaking intelligibly, are more likely to be associated with psychiatric causes.

Spiers et al. (1985); Trimble (2000).

Treatable Causes of Delirium and Dementia

Toxic	Metabolic	Infectious	Inflammatory	Other
Alcohol-associated dementia	Vitamin B_{12} or folate deficiency	Bacterial meningitis (chronic or partially treated)	Demyelinating disease (e.g., multiple sclerosis)	Psychiatric Bipolar disorder Depression Psychosis
Heavy metals (arsenic, lead, mercury, manganese)	Thyroid disease (hypo- or hyper-)	Fungal or tuberculous meningitis	Limbic encephalitis	Hydrocephalus (obstructive or normal pressure)
Histiotoxic anoxia (carbon monoxide, cyanide)	Thiamine or niacin deficiency	Neurosyphilis	Lupus erythematosus	Neoplastic Carcinomatosis Meningeal lesions
Drugs Sedatives, Antidepressants, Antiarrhythmics, Anticonvulsants, Digitalis, Anticholinergics	Chronic hypertension Hypopituitarism Hypercalcemia Hyper- and hyponatremia Hypoglycemia Hypercapnia Parathyroid disease Porphyria Cushing's disease Uremia Wilson's disease	Viral encephalitis (herpes, HIV) Brain abscess Parasitic encephalitis Systemic infection in elderly or cognitively compromised Whipple's disease of CNS	Sarcoidosis Sjögren's syndrome Behçet's syndrome	Primary tumors Metastatic lesions Remote effects Epilepsy Sleep apnea

A subset of patients seen for dementia will have a treatable cause. Some of the more common "reversible" causes include structural brain lesions (subdural hematomas, hydrocephalus), endocrine and nutritional deficits (thyroid, B_{12}), and the pseudodementia of depression. Therefore, the minimal workup of dementia of unknown cause should include neuroimaging, complete serum chemistries and CBC, thyroid function tests, B_{12} and folate levels, and neurobehavioral testing. See also *Acute Confusion*, in Chapter 1. Fleming, Adams, and Petersen (1995).

Neurodegenerative Causes of Dementia

Disease	Clinical Features	Pathology	Genetics
Alzheimer's disease	Progressive loss of orientation and memory. Deficits in language, visual, spatial function, and praxis. Executive dysfunction and eventual loss of ability to perform activities of daily living.	Neuritic plaques, neurofibrillary tangles, loss of synapses, neuronal cell loss, granulovacuolar degeneration, amyloid plaques, and amyloid angiopathy.	Familial cases: Chr. 21: amyloid precursor protein Chr. 14: presenilin 1 Chr. 1: presenilin 2 Sporadic risk factor: Chr. 19: apolipoprotein ε4
Frontotemporal lobar degeneration	Alteration of personality and social conduct with inertia, or social disinhibition and distractibility and relative sparing of memory. Subtypes: progressive aphasia, semantic dementia, frontotemporal dementia.	Two main histologic types: 1. Frontal lobe degeneration type: prominent microvacuolar change without specific histologic features. 2. Pick type: severe astrocytic gliosis with or without ballooned cells and inclusion bodies.	Familial cases: Chr. 17q21-23: mutations in the *tau* gene; also some families with linkage to Chr. 3
Huntington's disease	Chorea, executive dysfunction, psychosis, emotional lability.	Neuronal loss in the caudate and putamen; loss of GABA and multiple other neurotransmitters.	Chr. 4p16.3: CAG repeat in the *Huntingtin* gene
Dementia with Lewy bodies	Parkinsonism, visual hallucinations, fluctuations in cognition.	Lewy bodies in the brainstem, basal forebrain, limbic structures, and neocortex.	
Parkinson's disease	Rigidity, postural instability, resting tremor, psychomotor slowing, executive dysfunction, delusions and hallucinations.	Neuronal loss in the substantia nigra pars compacta, Lewy bodies in the substantia nigra and other brainstem nuclei.	Some familial cases linked to mutation of the *α-synuclein* gene on Chr. 4q21-22

Progressive supranuclear palsy (PSP)	Parkinsonism, ophthalmoplegia, psycho-motor slowing, axial rigidity, pseudobulbar palsy	Degeneration and neurofibrillary tangles in nucleus basalis, pallidum, subthalamic nucleus, superior colliculi, substantia nigra, and other brainstem nuclei.	*Tau* gene is a candidate
Spinocerebellar degeneration	Later development of psychomotor slowing, executive dysfunction, emotional lability in setting of ataxia, ophthalmoplegia, pyramidal weakness, and peripheral neuropathy.	Pathology variable, even within families, with degeneration in cerebellum, spinal cord, basal ganglia, and cerebral cortex.	CAG repeats in *SCA1* (Chr. 6p) *SCA2* (Chr. 12q); *SCA3* (Chr. 14q) Note other SCA gene syndromes not associated with dementia
Cortical-basal ganglionic degeneration	Akinetic rigid syndrome, apraxia, cortical sensory dysfunction and "alien-hand" syndrome (involuntary purposeful unilateral hand movements).	Neuronal degeneration in pre- and postcentral cortical areas, basal ganglia, substantia nigra. Achromatic neural inclusions in the cortex, thalamus, subthalamic nucleus, red nucleus, and substantia nigra.	

GABA: γ-aminobutyric acid.

Blacker and Tanzi (1998); Geldmacher and Whitehouse (1996); McKeith et al. (1996); Neary et al. (1998).

Cortical vs. Subcortical Dementia

Function	Cortical Dementia	Subcortical Dementia
Psychomotor speed	Normal	Slowed
Language	Involved	Spared
Memory		
Recall	Impaired	Impaired
Recognition	Impaired	Spared
Remote	Temporal gradient present	Temporal gradient absent
Executive function	Less involved	More involved
Depression	Less common	More common
Apathy	Less common	More common
Motor system	Spared until late	Involved early
Localization	Cerebral cortex	Subcortical structures and dorsolateral prefrontal cortex projecting to the head of the caudate
Examples	Alzheimer's disease, Pick's disease	Huntington's disease, HIV encephalopathy, lacunar state, normal pressure hydrocephalus

Dementia may be divided into descriptive categories of *cortical* and *subcortical*. Cortical dementia is characterized by prominent deficits in memory, language, and other higher cognitive functions. Subcortical dementia is distinguished by marked apathy, slowed thinking, and poor recall. Note that these terms do not strictly describe the underlying anatomic sites of pathology; both cortical and subcortical dementias can affect diffuse areas of the brain.

Cummings and Trimble (1995).

Vascular Causes of Dementia

Multiinfarct dementia

Caused by multiple large cerebral emboli of cardiogenic origin or arising from athero-sclerotic plaques in the walls of the aorto-cephalic arterial tree. Multiple infarctions result from occlusions of main trunks or branches of anterior, middle, and posterior cerebral arteries, producing cortical deficits characterized by aphasia, dyslexia, agraphia, amnesia, agnosia, inattention, and impersistence. Occlusion of internal carotid and/or vertebral arteries may cause watershed ischemia between major vascular territories, resulting in cortical plus white matter infarctions with similar cognitive impairments.

Strategically placed infarcts

May be single or multiple and due to any cause that involves the thalamus or frontal white matter, basal ganglia, or angular gyrus that results in impairment of memory or judgment, dysnomia, agraphia, alexia, dyscalculia, constructional apraxia, or disorientation in space or body parts.

Subcortical vascular dementia

Multiple subcortical lacunar infarcts due to occlusion of penetrating arterioles and lenticulostriate arteries resulting in apathy, slowness of mental processing, psychomotor retardation, bradykinesia, disorientation, impaired memory and attention, perse-veration, impersistence, and difficulty shifting from one set to another. Lacunar infarcts are the most common type of vascular dementia. 23% of patients with lacunar infarcts confirmed by CT or MRI will develop dementia within 4 years. See also *Cortical vs. Subcortical Dementia.*

Binswanger's subcortical arteriosclerotic leukoencephalopathy

Brought about by multiple cumulative occlusions of deep penetrating arterioles supplying white matter, resulting in more severe patterns of subcortical dementia, with abulia, incontinence, and limb rigidity. Criteria for clinical diagnosis:

1. Presence of associated risk factors for stroke (hypertension, amyloid angiopathy, antiphospholipid antibodies) or a family history of stroke, as is seen in CADASIL or in familial amyloid angiopathies and coagulopathies. See also *Inherited Causes of Stroke,* in Chapter 2.

2. Focal ischemic lacunar lesions of white matter that are often confluent by neuro-imaging.

3. Age between 55 and 75 years (may be late 30s or early 40s in CADASIL).

4. Subacute onset of focal neurological signs with progression over days, weeks, or rarely years, with pyramidal, extrapyramidal, and pseudobulbar signs plus abulia with both cognitive and neurobehavioral deterioration.

5. The greater the number of neurological signs, the more likely is the diagnosis of Binswanger's disease to be correct.

CADASIL: cerebral autosomal dominant arteriopathy with subcortical infarcts and leukoen-cephalopathy.

Loeb and Meyer (1996).

Neurologic Disorders with Psychiatric Symptoms

Disorder	Depression	Mania	Psychosis
Stroke (left hemisphere)	Severe psychomotor retardation		Particularly involving temporal lobe (Wernicke's area)
Stroke (right hemisphere)		Particularly in patients with family history of psychiatric disease	
Parkinson's disease	Anxiety common	After dopaminergic therapy	After dopaminergic therapy
Huntington's disease	Suicide is common	Episodes of elevated mood or irritability	Delusions
Epilepsy	Frequency of suicide increased	During perictal periods	Particularly with temporal lobe focus
Traumatic brain injury	More likely in patients with history of psychiatric disorder or substance abuse	More likely in patients with right hemisphere contusions	Particularly during phase of posttraumatic encephalopathy
Multiple sclerosis	Depression not related to degree of disability	Hypomanic or cyclothymic presentation	Delusions
Alzheimer's disease	Dysthymia common, but major depressive episodes rare		Paranoid delusions most common
Vascular dementia	Common in lacunar state and Binswanger's disease		Delusions
Frontotemporal dementias		Hyperirritability, hypomanic overactivity	Delusions
Neurosyphilis		Overactivity, lack of awareness of deficits	

Dementia with Lewy bodies	Visual hallucinations common
Creutzfeldt-Jakob disease	Delusions
Vitamin B_{12} deficiency	Grandiose delusions
Inborn disorders of metabolism	Metachromatic leukodystrophy, adrenoleukodystrophy, GM_2 gangliosidosis, neuronal ceroid lipofuscinosis mitochondrial encephalopathy

Cummings and Trimble (1995).

Neurobehavioral Syndromes

Syndrome	Features	Localization
Dorsolateral prefrontal (pseudodepressed)	Impairment of executive functions, including abstract reasoning, problem solving, judgment, set shifting, and divided and sustained attention	Dorsolateral prefrontal cortex, caudate, globus pallidus, thalamus
Orbitofrontal (pseudopsychopathic)	Disinhibition, lack of social conventions, impulsive, labile and irritable mood, hypomania/mania, impaired olfactory recognition; intellectual skills spared	Lateral orbital cortex, ventral caudate, globus pallidus, thalamus
Medial frontal (apathetic)	Emotional: unmotivated, poor initiation, lack of goal formation; Motor: does not engage, or participate (akinetic mutism); Cognitive: loss of planning, generative thought, slow cognition	Anterior cingulate cortex, nucleus accumbens, globus pallidus, thalamus
Kluver-Bucy syndrome	Hypersexuality, loss of fear and aggression, hyperorality and hypermetamorphosis (excessive attention to external stimuli)	Bilateral temporal lobe dysfunction
Geschwind syndrome	Hypergraphia, interpersonal "viscosity," circumstantial speech, hyposexuality, hyperreligiosity	Temporal lobe epilepsy
Angular gyrus syndrome	All elements of Gerstmann syndrome plus constructional deficits, alexia, anomia, ideomotor apraxia, verbal memory disturbance (often mistaken for Alzheimer's disease)	Left angular gyrus (larger lesion than that producing Gerstmann syndrome)
Gerstmann syndrome	Agraphia, acalculia, right-left disorientation, finger agnosia	Left angular gyrus (only if all elements present)
Anton's syndrome	Cortical blindness with denial of blindness	Bilateral optic radiations or occipital cortex
Balint's syndrome	Simultanagnosia (inability to perceive more than one part of the visual field at a time), optic ataxia (errors in reaching for seen objects), and optic apraxia (inability to voluntarily shift gaze)	Bilateral parietal-occipital junction lesions

Chow and Cummings (1999); Cummings and Trimble (1995); Damasio and Anderson (1993).

Drawing in Patients with Right Parietal Lobe Lesions

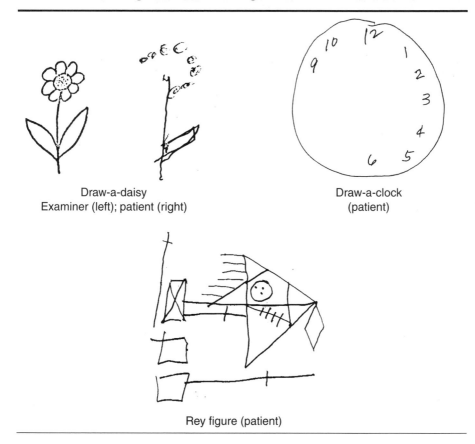

Draw-a-daisy
Examiner (left); patient (right)

Draw-a-clock
(patient)

Rey figure (patient)

Patients with right parietal lobe lesions often show striking neglect on the left side of their environment. This is exemplified in the drawing samples here. The patient's copy of the Rey figure, daisy, and clock all have relatively poor detail drawn on the left side of the figures.

Rey figure—Reprinted with permission from Kaplan E. A process approach to neuropsychological assessment. In: Boll T, Bryant BK, eds. *Clinical Neuropsychology and Brain Function.* Washington, D.C.: American Psychological Association; 1988:161. **Daisy figure**—Reprinted with permission from Heilman KM, Watson RT, Valenstein E. Neglect and related disorders. In: Heilman KM, Valenstein E, eds. *Clinical Neuropsychology.* New York: Oxford University Press; 1985:246. **Clock figure**—Reprinted with permission from Heilman KM, Watson RT, Valenstein E. Neglect: Clinical and anatomic aspects. In: Feinberg TE, Farah MJ, eds. *Behavioral Neurology and Neuropsychology.* New York: McGraw-Hill; 1997:314.

REFERENCES

Benson DF. Aphasia. In: Heilman KM, Valenstein E, eds. *Clinical Neuropsychology.* New York: Oxford University Press; 1993:17–36.

Benton A, Tranel D. Visuoperceptual, visuospatial, and visuoconstructive disorders. In: Heilman KM, Valenstein E, eds. *Clinical Neuropsychology.* New York: Oxford University Press; 1993:165–213.

Blacker D, Tanzi RE. The genetics of Alzheimer disease. *Arch Neurol.* 1998;55:294–296.

Chow TW, Cummings JL. Frontal-subcortical circuits. In: Miller BL, Cummings JL, eds. *The Human Frontal Lobes: Functions and Disorders.* New York: Guilford Press; 1999:3–26.

Cummings JL, Trimble MR. *Concise Guide to Neuropsychiatry and Behavioral Neurology.* Washington, D.C.: American Psychiatric Press: 1995:38–44.

Damasio AR. Disorders of complex visual processing, agnosias, achromatopsia, Balint's syndrome and related difficulties of orientation and construction. In: Mesulam M-M, ed. *Principles of Behavioral Neurology.* Philadelphia: F.A. Davis Co.; 1985.

Damasio AR, Anderson SW. The frontal lobes. In: Heilman KM, Valenstein E, eds. *Clinical Neuropsychology.* New York: Oxford University Press; 1993:409–460.

Fleming KC, Adams AC, Petersen RC. Dementia: Diagnosis and evaluation. *Mayo Clin Proc.* 1995;70:1093–1107.

Geldmacher DS, Whitehouse PJ. Evaluation of dementia. *New Engl J Med.* 1996;335:330–336.

Heilman KM, Watson RT, Valenstein E. Neglect and related disorders. In: Heilman KM, Valenstein E, eds. *Clinical Neuropsychology.* New York: Oxford University Press; 1985:246.

Heilman KM, Rothi LJG. Apraxia. In: Heilman KM, Valenstein E, eds. *Clinical Neuropsychology.* New York: Oxford University Press; 1993: 141–163.

Heilman KM, Watson RT, Valenstein E. Neglect and related disorders. In: Heilman KM, Valenstein E, eds. *Clinical Neuropsychology.* New York: Oxford University Press; 1993:279–336.

Heilman KM, Watson RT, Valenstein E. Neglect: Clinical and anatomic aspects. In: Feinberg TE, Farah MJ, eds. *Behavioral Neurology and Neuropsychology.* New York: McGraw-Hill; 1997:314.

Kaplan E. A process approach to neuropsychological assessment. In: Boll T, Bryant BK, eds. *Clinical Neuropsychology and Brain Function.* Washington, D.C.: American Psychological Association; 1988:161.

Loeb C, Meyer JS. Vascular dementia: still a debatable entity? *J Neurol Sci.* 1996;143:31–40.

McKeith IG, Galasko D, Kosaka K, et al. Consensus guidelines for the clinical and pathologic diagnosis of dementia with Lewy bodies (DLB):

Report of the consortium on DLB international workshop. *Neurology.* 1996;47:1113–1124.

Mesulam M-M. A cortical network for directed attention and unilateral neglect. *Ann Neurol.* 1981;10:309–325.

Neary D, Snoden JS, Gustafson L, et al. Frontotemporal lobar degeneration: A consensus on clinical diagnostic criteria. *Neurology.* 1998;51: 1546–1554.

Spiers PA, Schomer DL, Blume HW, et al. Temporolimbic epilepsy and behavior. In: Mesulam M-M, ed. *Principles of Behavioral Neurology.* Philadelphia: F.A. Davis Co.; 1985:289–326.

Trimble, MR. Depression and psychosis in neurological practice. In: Bradley WG, Daroff RB, Fenichel GM, Marsden CD, eds. *Neurology in Clinical Practice.* 3rd ed. Boston: Butterworth-Heinemann; 2000: 105–115.

Wilson BA. *Rehabilitation of Memory.* New York: Guilford Press; 1987: 15–36.

12

Neuroimaging

Joseph D. Pinter and Jong M. Rho

Neuroimaging Signal Characteristics

Tissue	CT	T1WI	T2WI
Bone	Bright	Dark	Dark
Air	Dark	Dark	Dark
Fat	Dark	Bright	Bright*
Water (CSF, edema, infarct)	Dark	Dark	Bright
Brain**			
Gray matter	Dark	Dark	Bright
White matter	Bright	Bright	Dark

*Fat is less bright on T2WI than T1WI and variable depending on the specific T2WI sequence.

**Brain is intermediate in signal intensity compared to the other entities listed here, but gray and white matter will be relatively dark or bright (compared to each other) depending on the imaging modality.

CT (computed tomography) is based on differential absorption of X-ray beams by different body tissues.

MRI (magnetic resonance imaging) is accomplished by placing body tissues in a fixed magnetic field and applying radio-frequency (RF) pulses, then measuring the signal generated as the tissue releases the energy absorbed and returns to longitudinal (spin-lattice) and transverse (spin-spin) magnetic equilibrium. Some commonly used imaging modalities and parameters are:

TR (repetition time): the time between successive RF pulses.

TE (echo time): the time between RF pulse and signal measurement.

T1 (T1 relaxation time): the time to return to longitudinal equilibrium (constant for a tissue).

T2 (T2 relaxation time): the time to return to transverse equilibrium (resting spin-spin interactions).

T1WI (short TR/short TE): tissues or substances with short T1 (including paramagnetic materials like gadolinium) appear bright on T1WI because more recovery occurs by the time the signal is measured. T1WI gives an "anatomical" picture of the brain, in which gray matter is dark and white matter bright. T1WI is also used for gadolinium- (contrast-) enhanced scans.

T2WI (long TR/long TE): tissues with long T2 appear bright on T2WI. T2WI gives a "pathological" view of the brain, in which edema-causing processes such as infarcts appear bright.

FLAIR (fluid-attenuated inversion recovery): nulls out the signal for CSF, therefore is more sensitive for edema, early demyelination or infarct, and cysts or low-grade tumors; it is useful for evaluating hippocampal pathology in temporal lobe epilepsy.

Woodruff (1993:33–70).

Neuroradiologic Anatomy

Imaging planes and major structures

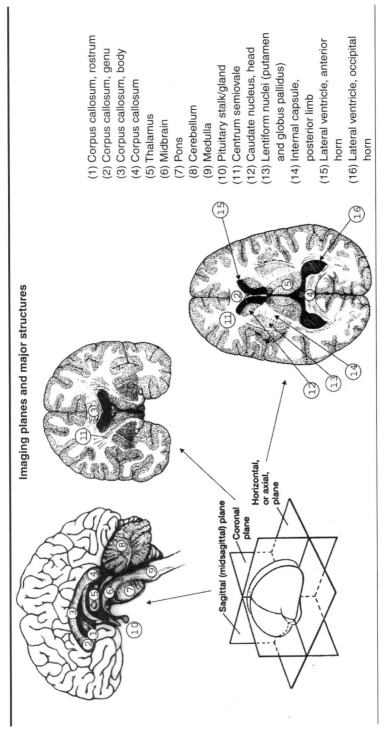

(1) Corpus callosum, rostrum
(2) Corpus callosum, genu
(3) Corpus callosum, body
(4) Corpus callosum
(5) Thalamus
(6) Midbrain
(7) Pons
(8) Cerebellum
(9) Medulla
(10) Pituitary stalk/gland
(11) Centrum semiovale
(12) Caudate nucleus, head
(13) Lentiform nuclei (putamen and globus pallidus)
(14) Internal capsule, posterior limb
(15) Lateral ventricle, anterior horn
(16) Lateral ventricle, occipital horn

Sagittal (midsagittal) plane
Coronal plane
Horizontal, or axial, plane

Brain diagrams modified with permission from Atlas SW. *Magnetic Resonance Imaging of the Brain and Spine on CD-ROM.* Philadelphia: Lippincott-Raven Publishers; 1998. Imaging plane reprinted with permission from Waxman SG. *Correlative Neuroanatomy.* New York: McGraw-Hill; 1996:299.

Angiographic Anatomy

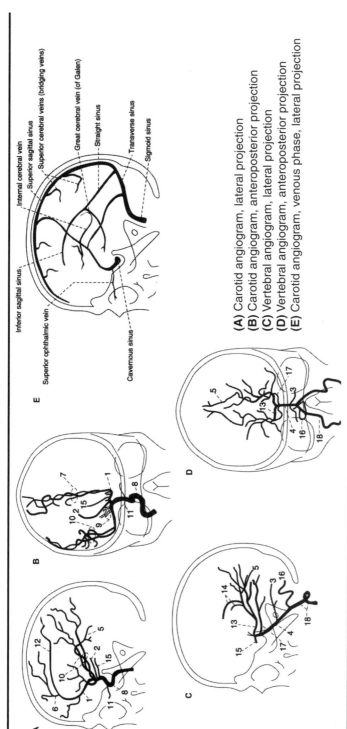

(A) Carotid angiogram, lateral projection
(B) Carotid angiogram, anteroposterior projection
(C) Vertebral angiogram, lateral projection
(D) Vertebral angiogram, anteroposterior projection
(E) Carotid angiogram, venous phase, lateral projection

(1) Anterior cerebral artery, (2) anterior choroidal artery, (3) anterior inferior cerebellar artery, (4) basilar artery, (5) calcarine artery (of posterior cerebral), (6) callosomarginal artery (of anterior cerebral), (7) callosomarginal and pericallosal arteries (of anterior cerebral), (8) internal carotid artery, (9) lateral striate arteries (of middle cerebral), (10) middle cerebral artery, (11) ophthalmic artery, (12) pericallosal artery (of anterior cerebral), (13) posterior cerebral artery, (14) posterior choroidal arteries (of posterior cerebral), (15) posterior communicating artery, (16) posterior inferior cerebellar artery, (17) superior cerebellar artery, (18) vertebral artery.

Reprinted with permission from Fix JD. *High-Yield Neuroanatomy*. Philadelphia: Lippincott Williams & Wilkins; 2000:19–20.

Vascular Territories of the Brain

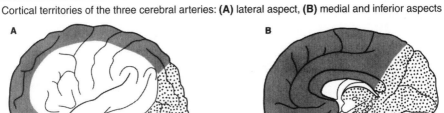

Cortical territories of the three cerebral arteries: **(A)** lateral aspect, **(B)** medial and inferior aspects

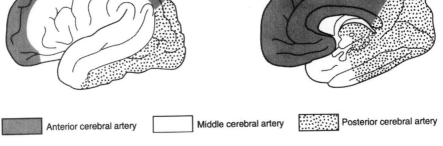

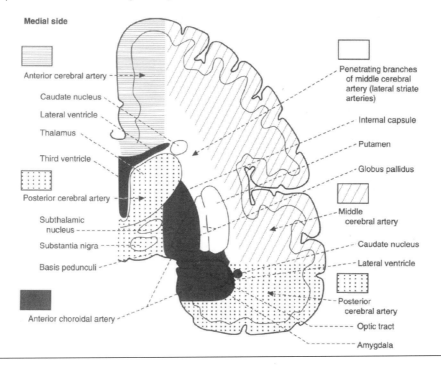

Schematic drawing of a coronal section through the cerebral hemisphere at the level of the internal capsule and thalamus showing the major vascular territories.

Neuroimaging of Ischemic Stroke

Time	CT	MRI (T1WI)	MRI (T2WI)
Immediate (minutes)	Normal	Absence of flow void in affected vessel (thrombus) Gadolinium (+) intravascular in 75% (slow flow)	Absence of flow void in affected vessel
Hyperacute (<6 hr)	Normal (25–50%) Hyperdensity in affected artery (thrombus) in 25–50% Mild parenchymal hypodensity	Sulcal effacement (early mass effect) Loss of gray-white differentiation	May be normal
Early acute (6–24 hr)	Sulcal effacement (early mass effect) Loss of gray/white differentiation Low density in basal ganglia	↑ mass effect Meningeal enhancement over affected area	↑ signal in affected area
Late acute (1–3 days)	Wedge of low density in arterial distribution, affecting both gray and white matter ↑ mass effect	↑ mass effect Decreased meningeal enhancement Early enhancement of parenchyma	Hyperintense
Early subacute (4–7 days)	Persistent mass effect or edema ± gyral enhancement with contrast	Parenchymal enhancement with gadolinium	Subcortical hyperintensity (15%) Acute wallerian degeneration (increased signal in descending corticospinal tracts)
Late subacute (1–8 weeks)	Resolving mass effect Persistent gyral enhancement	Mass effect resolves	↓ in areas of abnormal hyperintense signal
Chronic (months to years)	Atrophy or encephalomalacia ↑ size of sulci/ventricles No enhancement	Volume loss Atrophy Wallerian degeneration (volume loss)	Encephalomalacia

CT is initially relatively insensitive to ischemic changes, compared with MRI, but is valuable in evaluating for hemorrhage or mass effect when deciding whether to anticoagulate. Early ischemic changes are seen more easily on T2WI as hyperintense foci. Diffusion-weighted MRI (DWI) is the most sensitive for very early change, showing hyperintensity within an hour in regions of decreased water diffusion. The imaging findings in this table reflect only general changes seen with ischemia and infarction and do not differentiate between thrombotic and embolic causes. Note also that a fraction of ischemic stroke will undergo minor degrees of subacute hemorrhagic conversion; the appearance of this hemorrhage will vary on MRI depending on its age. See *Neuroimaging of Hemorrhage.*

Osborne and Tong (1996:373–385).

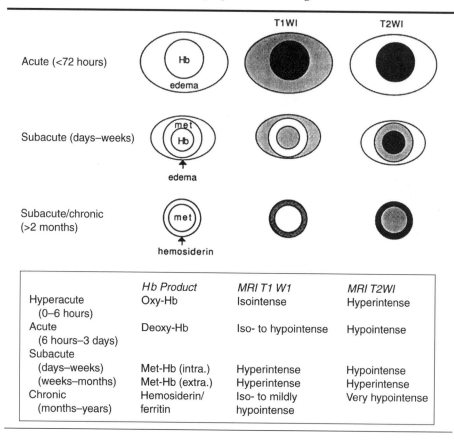

	Hb Product	MRI T1 W1	MRI T2WI
Hyperacute (0–6 hours)	Oxy-Hb	Isointense	Hyperintense
Acute (6 hours–3 days)	Deoxy-Hb	Iso- to hypointense	Hypointense
Subacute			
(days–weeks)	Met-Hb (intra.)	Hyperintense	Hypointense
(weeks–months)	Met-Hb (extra.)	Hyperintense	Hyperintense
Chronic (months–years)	Hemosiderin/ ferritin	Iso- to mildly hypointense	Very hypointense

Hemorrhage visualized on MRI undergoes a complex series of signal changes depending on the age of the bleed. These changes are due to the progressive conversion of hemoglobin (Hb) contained in RBCs to a series of degradation products, each of which has differing signal characteristics. Initially, oxygenated Hb (Oxy-Hb) appears bright on T2WI largely due to the water content of extravasated blood. RBCs then rapidly become desaturated, and the resulting deoxy-Hb is apparent as a marked hypointensity on T2WI. Deoxy-Hb is then converted to met-Hb over several days, first within RBCs (intracellular met-Hb), in a process that begins at the periphery of the hemorrhage and gradually moves centripetally. This causes a ring of hyperintensity on T1WI that moves inward. As RBCs lyse and release met-Hb (extracellular met-Hb), its signal on T2WI changes. Over months, degradation of met-Hb liberates iron that is stored as hemosiderin and ferritin. This produces the typical picture of chronic hemorrhage, with a core of mixed signal intensity on T2WI, surrounded by a rim of very hypointense signal.

Note that for detection of acute hemorrhage (e.g., subarachnoid hemorrhage), CT remains the study of choice.

Figure modified with permission from Lufkin RB. *The MRI Manual.* Chicago: Year Book Medical Publishers; 1990:38.

Neuroimaging Features of CNS Infections

Meningitis	Often normal CT and MRI but can see dural, leptomeningeal, and ependymal enhancement on T1WI. Tuberculous meningitis tends to produce marked enhancement of basilar cisterns.
Abscess	Ring-enhancing lesion on T1WI. Smooth capsule of low T2WI signal (hypointense)—thicker on side toward gray matter—with surrounding vasogenic edema (hypointense on T1, hyperintense on T2). Seen mainly in temporal, frontal, and parietal lobes.
Encephalitis	CT initially normal or only subtly hypodense lesion with mild mass effect. MRI shows early gyral edema on T1WI (with patchy gyral enhancement ± petechial hemorrhage late in course). On T2WI, areas of hyperintensity are seen which can look like infarct (but do not respect vascular boundaries), tumor, or abscess.
	HSV I is the most common cause of diagnosable encephalitis cases in adults. It involves mainly limbic areas (temporal lobes, insular cortex, subfrontal area, cingulate gyri). Often initially unilateral, later bilateral.
Fungal infection	CNS involvement by fungal organisms produces a nonspecific meningitis (often basilar) or meningoencephalitis in most cases. Notable exceptions include Aspergillosis and Mucormycosis, which can invade the CNS from the sinuses.
Parasitic infection	
Toxoplasmosis	Ring-enhancing 1–3 cm diameter lesion(s). Hypodense on CT, hypointense on T1WI, hyperintense on T2WI. Most common opportunistic infection in people with AIDS, although appearance can be mimicked by CNS lymphoma.
Neurocysticercosis	Imaging findings depend on stage of parasite life cycle. As cysts die there is incomplete ring enhancement and edema, which later becomes a classic ring-enhancing cystic lesion, often with a central nodule (the scolex of the parasite). In the final (nodular) stage, lesions are calcified with no edema or enhancement. Lesions most often are at gray/white junction, reflecting hematogenous spread. Most common parasitic infection among immunocompetent patients, who usually present with seizure or headache.

Castillo (1999); Osborne and Tong (1996:442–455).

Neuroimaging Features of Cerebrovascular Malformations

	Arteriovenous Malformation	Venous Angioma	Cavernous Angioma	Capillary Telangiectasia
CT unenhanced	Irregular Hyperdense Calcification Atrophy	Solitary Dense Tubular structure	Solitary or multiple dense lesions; may contain calcification	Solitary density in pons
CT enhanced	Serpentine enhancement Draining veins	Transcerebral vein and caput medusae	Minimal to no enhancement	Minimal to no enhancement
MRI T1WI	Multiple tubular flow voids	Solitary tubular flow void	Focus of heterogeneous signal May be multiple No flow effects	Like cavernous angioma but solitary and in pons
MRI T2WI	Flow void	Flow void	Complex heterogeneous signal surrounded by rim of hypointensity; may be multiple	Like cavernous angioma but solitary and in pons
Angiography Arterial phase	Hypertrophied arterial feeders Nidus Early venous phase	Normal	Normal	Normal
Venous phase	Multiple ectatic early draining veins	Solitary transcerebral vein Caput medusae	Normal or may see late capillary blush	Normal

Cerebrovascular malformations are developmental abnormalities of brain blood vessels present in 4% of the general population. Arteriovenous malformations (AVMs) are direct connections of arterial and venous channels with no intervening capillary bed; they have a significant risk of bleeding, ~3-4% per year. While the second commonest vascular malformation, AVMs are the most likely to be symptomatic. In contrast, venous angiomas are the most common brain vascular malformation but have little or no risk of bleeding. They may be identified on angiography by enlarged medullary veins that drain into a solitary transcerebral vein ("caput medusae"). Cavernous angiomas are the third most common (10%) intracranial vascular malformation and are multiple in a third of cases. These lesions are at risk of bleeding, and MRI usually shows a hypointense rim on T2WI, which represents hemosiderin from prior hemorrhage. Capillary telangiectasias are solitary lesions, usually found in the pons. Their risk of bleeding is low, and they usually are an incidental finding on neuroimaging.

Modified with permission from Woodruff WW. *Fundamentals of Neuroimaging*. Philadelphia: W.B. Saunders Co.; 1993:158.

Neuroimaging of White Matter Disease

Vascular causes

Small vessel disease is the most common acquired white matter disorder. It appears as multiple small foci of increased T2WI signal in subcortical white matter, corona radiata, and basal ganglia, sometimes in setting of lacunar stroke. Its appearance overlaps with the dilated perivascular spaces seen with aging.

Demyelination

Multiple sclerosis (MS) In >85% patients, there are ovoid periventricular lesions, with their long axis perpendicular to the lateral ventricles, most evident on T2WI. Of MS patients, 50–90% have lesions within the corpus callosum. Enhancement, often in a ring pattern, is seen with active lesions. Usually multiple lesions are seen, often with brainstem, cerebellar, and spinal involvement. FLAIR is very sensitive for periventricular lesions.

Acute disseminated encephalomyelitis (ADEM) Lesions similar to (and sometimes indistinguishable from) MS but more often involving centrum semiovale and deep gray nuclei. Lesions are bilateral, asymmetric, and often enhance. Illness usually is monophasic and follows by 1–3 weeks a nonspecific viral infection or vaccination.

Progressive multifocal leukoencephalopathy (PML) Same lesion appearance on CT, T1WI, and T2WI as MS and ADEM, with single or multiple scattered lesions, most commonly occipitoparietal, that may become confluent late. Notably, these lesions do not enhance or show mass effect. Seen primarily in immunosuppressed patients or those with AIDS.

Leukodystrophies

Metachromatic leukodystrophy (MLD), adrenoleukodystrophy (ALD), Krabbe's disease. These diseases show nonspecific atrophy of primarily deep white matter, sparing subcortical white matter.

> *MLD:* Bilateral, symmetric high T2WI signal in periventricular white matter, initially patchy, later confluent.

> *ALD:* Predominantly parieto-occipital white matter (typically including splenium of corpus callosum), progression from central to peripheral, posterior to anterior. CT may reveal punctate calcification; advancing rim enhances with contrast.

> *Krabbe's:* Parietal region, optic pathways often affected first, with nonspecific confluent symmetric hyperintensity in deep cerebral and cerebellar white matter on T2WI.

Alexander's (A), Canavan's (C), Pelizaeus-Merzbacher (P-M) diseases These diseases tend to affect peripheral (subcortical) white matter early. Macrocephaly is seen in both A and C.

> *A:* Frontal deep and subcortical white matter. Basal ganglia may enhance with contrast.

> *C:* Diffuse involvement of all white matter, including subcortical U fibers (similar to *P-M*).

> *P-M:* Patchy, variable, with severe cases showing near-total lack of myelination in deep and superficial white matter (newborn appearance); diffuse atrophy.

Radiation or chemotherapy (e.g., methotrexate, cyclosporine)

Such treatment also can lead to focal, or often diffuse, white matter T2WI hyperintensities. Combination can lead to severe necrotizing leukoencephalopathy.

CADASIL (cerebral autosomal dominant arteriopathy with subcortical infarcts and leukoencephalopathy)

Rare, inherited disorder with characteristic MRI findings even when presymptomatic: extensive symmetric increased T2WI signal in periventricular and lobar white matter, mostly in anterior temporal regions. External > internal capsule involvement, absence of cortical lesions, sparing of subcortical U fibers. Small, well-delineated deep lesions with decreased T1WI and increased T2WI consistent with lacunar infarctions of the basal ganglia and thalami.

See also *White Matter Lesions on Neuroimaging: Multiple Sclerosis vs. Vascular Etiologies* and *White Matter Lesions on Neuroimaging: Multiple Sclerosis vs. Infectious, Inflammatory, and Metabolic Disorders,* in Chapter 3.

Osborne and Tong (1996:517–527, 545–559, 668); Loevner (1999); Castillo (1999:140–160); Greenberg (1999).

Neuroimaging of Myelination in Infants

Anatomic region	Age of Appearance of "Adult" Pattern	
	T1WI (bright)	T2WI (dark)
Middle cerebellar peduncle	Birth	Birth–2 mon
Cerebellar white matter	Birth–4 mon	3–5 mon
Posterior limb, internal capsule		
Anterior portion	Birth–1 mon	4–7 mon
Posterior portion	Birth	Birth–2 mon
Anterior limb, internal capsule	2–3 mon	7–11 mon
Genu, corpus callosum	4–6 mon	5–8 mon
Splenium, corpus callosum	3–4 mon	4–6 mon
Occipital white matter		
Central	3–5 mon	9–14 mon
Peripheral	4–7 mon	11–15 mon
Frontal white matter		
Central	3–6 mon	11–16 mon
Peripheral	7–11 mon	14–18 mon
Centrum semiovale	2–6 mon	7–11 mon

In early infancy, the appearance of brain white matter on MRI is the opposite of the adult pattern, with white matter appearing relatively dark on T1WI and bright on T2WI. This is due to the incomplete myelination of axons. The situation gradually transforms into the adult pattern (bright on T1WI and dark on T2WI) over the first 2 years, with different structures achieving myelination at different times. Some representative structures are listed here, in order of myelination. Myelination generally progresses (1) from caudad to cephalad, (2) from dorsal to ventral, (3) from central to peripheral. The changes in signal reflect mainly increased bound water in myelin, resulting in shortening of T1 (increased brightness on T1WI).

Although it is not clear why T1WI and T2WI myelination changes occur at different times, T1WI is more useful for assessing myelination in the first year.

Modified with permission from Barkovich AJ. *Pediatric Neuroimaging*. Philadelphia: Lippincott Williams & Wilkins; 2000:38.

Osborne and Tong (1996).

Neuroimaging Features of Neurocutaneous Disorders

Neurofibromatosis type 1 (NF1)

Single or multiple gliomas of the optic nerve and hemispheric visual pathways are a hallmark of this disease. Gliomas in other parts of the brain and spinal cord (usually low-grade astrocytomas) also occur. Peripheral nerve neurofibromas (e.g., of spinal nerve roots) are diagnostic. Of note, high-T2WI lesions are seen in 80% of children, commonly in basal ganglia, internal capsule, optic radiation, and brainstem/cerebellum. These lesions are of unknown clinical significance and usually regress after age 10.

Neurofibromatosis type 2 (NF2)

Brain lesions arise from brain and nerve coverings, producing schwannomas, meningiomas, and ependymomas. Bilateral vestibular nerve schwannomas (acoustic neuromas) are diagnostic, but schwannomas also can arise from other cranial nerves (such as V) and spinal nerve roots. Schwannomas are slightly hyperintense on T2WI. Meningiomas also frequently are seen, hypointense on T2WI, often multiple, and in atypical locations. Both enhance intensely. Spinal cord ependymomas are common, with meningiomas less common

Tuberous sclerosis (TS)

Over 95% of TS patients have benign brain hamartomas (tubers) on MRI. The most common tubers are subependymal nodules ("candle gutterings") protruding into ventricles, over 75% are calcified, and 30% enhance. Because of calcification (which increases with age), these periventricular lesions are easily identifiable on CT and appear as hypointense lesions on MRI. Cortical tubers are seen in 50% of patients, often bilaterally symmetric, with frontal > parietal > occipital > temporal lobe location. Of TS patients, 5–15% have subependymal giant cell astrocytomas—slow-growing, low-grade neoplasms most commonly located at the foramen of Monro. These tumors often are asymptomatic but sometimes cause hydrocephalus; growth on sequential imaging distinguishes these from more benign subependymal nodules.

Sturge-Weber syndrome

Encephalotrigeminal angiomatosis, a vascular disorder affecting brain, face (port-wine stain in V_1), and meninges, with occipitoparietal pial venous angioma that is ipsilateral to the facial skin lesion. CT shows "tram-track" calcifications in apposing gyri (often not seen before 2 years of age), which gradually atrophy. MRI may show hypointensity in areas of calcification. The pial angioma enhances strongly, as does the ipsilaterally enlarged choroid plexus. Also note the increased number and size of medullary, subependymal veins, providing collateral deep venous drainage for lack of cortical draining veins in area of pial angioma.

Von Hippel-Lindau (VHL) disease

Hemangioblastomas are the hallmark, with >50 % of VHL patients with one or more in brain or spinal cord: 90% are in posterior fossa (65% cerebellum, 20% brainstem), 10% in spinal cord. These are cystic, well-delineated masses, hyperintense on both T1WI and T2WI, with a mural nodule that enhances strongly. While these lesions are prone to hemorrhage, associated renal cell carcinoma, pheochromocytoma, and cystic disease of the liver, kidney and pancreas disorders cause significant morbidity and mortality.

Osborne and Tong (1996:163–175); Loevner (1999); Castillo (1999); Grossman and Yousem (1994).

Ultrasound Imaging of Neonatal Brain Hemorrhage

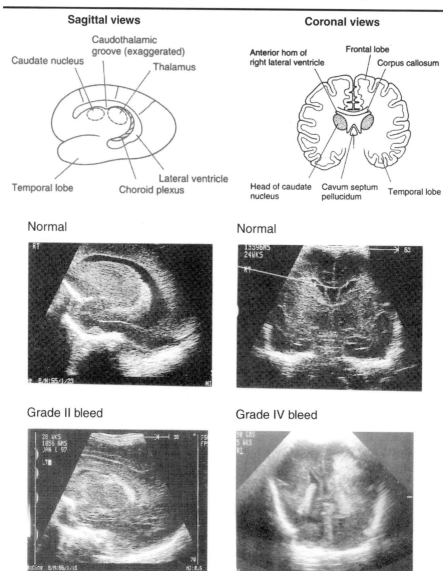

Intraventricular or periventricular hemorrhages (IVH or PVH) begin in the germinal matrix, abutting the lateral ventricles. They are most commonly identified by neonatal head ultrasound, which shows hyperechogenic areas of bleed, with or without large hypoechogenic ventricles reflecting hydrocephalus. Germinal matrix hemorrhage is an injury occurring in premature babies, and is unusual after 34 weeks of gestation due to the normal involution of the germinal matrix.

IVH grade	Definition
I	Germinal matrix bleed confined to subependymal region; no IVH
II	Extension of germinal matrix bleed into the ventricles, without ventricular enlargement (no hydrocephalus)
III	Extension into, and enlargement of ventricle(s); unilateral or bilateral hydrocephalus
IV	Involvement of periventricular brain parenchyma secondary to venous infarction, usually with IVH. Sometimes classified as "separate notation" to indicate that it is not an extension of IVH

Table reprinted with permission from Volpe JJ. *Neurology of the Newborn*. Philadelphia: W.B. Saunders Co.; 1995:403–463. Diagram reprinted with permission from Kirpalani H, Mernagh J, Gill G. *Imaging of the Newborn Baby*. London: Churchill Livingstone; 1999: 89–92.

REFERENCES

Atlas SW. *Magnetic Resonance Imaging of the Brain and Spine on CD-ROM.* Philadelphia: Lippincott-Raven Publishers; 1998.

Barkovich AJ. *Pediatric Neuroimaging.* Philadelphia: Lippincott Williams & Wilkins; 2000:38.

Castillo M. *Neuroradiology Companion: Methods, Guidelines and Imaging Fundamentals.* Philadelphia: Lippincott-Raven Publishers; 1999: 140–160.

Fix JD. *High-Yield Neuroanatomy.* Philadelphia: Lippincott Williams & Wilkins; 2000:19–20.

Greenberg J. *Neuroimaging: A Companion to Adams and Victor's Principles of Neurology.* New York: McGraw-Hill; 1999:97–98.

Grossman RI, Yousem DM. *Neuroradiology: The Requisites.* St. Louis: Mosby-Year Book; 1994:266–272.

Kirpalani H, Mernagh J, Gill G. *Imaging of the Newborn Baby.* London: Churchill Livingstone; 1999.

Loevner LA. *Case Review. Brain Imaging.* St. Louis: Mosby; 1999:58.

Lufkin RB. *The MRI Manual.* Chicago: Year Book Medical Publishers; 1990.

Osborne AG, Tong KA. *Handbook of Neuroradiology: Brain and Skull.* St. Louis: Mosby-Year Book; 1996:497–509.

Volpe JJ. *Neurology of the Newborn.* Philadelphia: W.B. Saunders Co.; 1995.

Waxman SG. *Correlative Neuroanatomy.* New York: McGraw-Hill; 1996: 299.

Woodruff WW. *Fundamentals of Neuroimaging.* Philadelphia: W.B. Saunders Co.; 1993:90–95.

Index

255